Medical Management of Eating Disorders

Third edition

Medical Management of Eating Disorders

Third edition

C. Laird Birmingham
University of British Columbia, Vancouver

Janet Treasure
Institute of Psychiatry, London

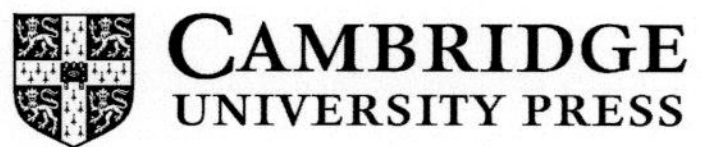

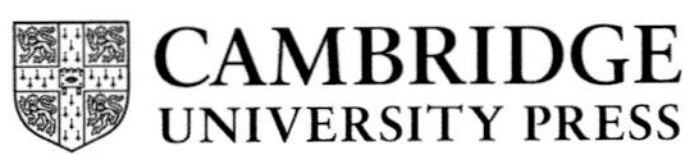

Shaftesbury Road, Cambridge CB2 8EA, United Kingdom

One Liberty Plaza, 20th Floor, New York, NY 10006, USA

477 Williamstown Road, Port Melbourne, VIC 3207, Australia

314–321, 3rd Floor, Plot 3, Splendor Forum, Jasola District Centre, New Delhi – 110025, India

103 Penang Road, #05–06/07, Visioncrest Commercial, Singapore 238467

Cambridge University Press is part of Cambridge University Press & Assessment, a department of the University of Cambridge.

We share the University's mission to contribute to society through the pursuit of education, learning and research at the highest international levels of excellence.

www.cambridge.org
Information on this title: www.cambridge.org/9781108465991

DOI: 10.1017/9781108618410

First published 2007
Second edition 2010
Third edition 2019

A catalogue record for this publication is available from the British Library

Library of Congress Cataloging-in-Publication data
Names: Birmingham, C. Laird (Carl Laird) author. | Treasure, Janet, author.
Title: Medical management of eating disorders / C. Laird Birmingham, University of British Columbia, Vancouver, Janet Treasure, Institute of Psychiatry, London.
Description: Third edition. | New York, NY : Cambridge University Press, [2019] | Includes index.
Identifiers: LCCN 2018051220 | ISBN 9781108465991 (pbk.)
Subjects: LCSH: Eating disorders. | Eating disorders–Complications.
Classification: LCC RC552.E18 B515 2019 | DDC 616.85/26–dc23
LC record available at https://lccn.loc.gov/2018051220

ISBN 978-1-108-46599-1 Paperback

Contents

Preface to Third Edition

'The medical management of eating disorders' has survived to its third edition because it has become a handbook referred to by eating disorder clinicians around the world. It is not a book that is generally read cover to cover. For this reason, The Third Edition of "The Medical Management of Eating Disorders" continues to have the information you need in each of the places you are likely to look for it. It is written entirely by Professors Treasure and Birmingham, who have used their own special skills, backgrounds, beliefs, and arguments to provide a balanced approach. However, no textbook can replace your own national guidelines, local laws, and unique approach to these puzzling diseases. The best approach may depend on the patient's belief system, the workings of the treatment team, financial resources, and the risk of the disease to the patient when you assess them.

We have prefaced some chapters with cases or questions to stimulate your interest. Chapters are followed by "Implications for health care professionals" to highlight the effect of the information on patterns of practice and "Patient Information" to help you to explain the information contained in the chapter to the patient.

The Third Edition of "The Medical Management of Eating Disorders" explains the *Diagnostic and Statistical Manual of Mental Disorders*, fifth edition, diagnosis of eating disorders and updates "Patient Self-Help" in the form of "Patient Self-Management." The chapter on mortality has been extended in scope and now focuses on how to decrease mortality.

We have updated treatment protocols, including those for magnesium replacement, constipation, and zinc supplementation, as well as the guidelines and warnings for the use of lisdexamfetamine dimesylate.

We hope that the third edition of "The Medical Management of Eating Disorders" will remain, or become, your handbook for the medical treatment of your patients with eating disorders.

C. Laird Birmingham & Janet Treasure

Preface to Second Edition

The 'Medical management of eating disorders' offers the reader a holistic approach to the management of eating disorders, in an easy to use handbook style. The reviews of the first edition of 'The medical management of eating disorders' were very positive – and made good suggestions for the book's improvement. To facilitate use of the information in the second edition, the format has been altered to that of a standard medical text: definitions and prevalence, cause, diagnosis and clinical features, complications, differential diagnosis, course and prognosis, and treatment. Obesity is discussed next, in Part 7. It is essential that health care professionals who treat eating disorders know the information presented about obesity, so they can understand and discuss these issues with their patients. All sections are followed by implications for health care professionals and patient information.

Janet Treasure has completely revised and updated the psychiatric management of eating disorders, for the second edition. There have been important advances in understanding causal mechanisms that are discussed. These include the importance to causation of the endophenotypes: social, emotional, perceptual and behavioural cognitive styles. This sets the stage for more biologically based diagnoses, which incorporate pathophysiology. Treatments can thereby be more closely tailored to the individual.

The second edition adds much new material, including: management of eating disorders with concurrent substance use, an approach to the differential diagnosis of eating disorders from the medical perspective, which laboratory tests to order and when to order them, when to perform and how to interpret the glucagon test, how to interpret the magnesium load test, how to diagnose the superior mesenteric artery syndrome, and how to decide whether the patient is at their physiologically normal weight.

The section on children and adolescents has been completely revised. The outline of history and physical examination has been improved. All major physical signs are now illustrated in colour photographs. The bibliography has been updated, and continues to be limited to only the most important references.

We would like to thank everyone who has adopted the first edition of "The medical management of eating disorders" as their handbook for the medical care of patients with eating disorders. We invite your feedback on the second edition!

C. Laird Birmingham & Janet Treasure

Preface to First Edition

This book is rather different from most written on eating disorders. Its sole purpose is to provide assistance to health professionals in the understanding, treatment, and management of patients with eating disorders, particularly that part of their treatment that is best described as medical. It is concerned primarily with anorexia nervosa (anorexia nervosa), as it is the member of this group of illnesses that has the most serious medical manifestations, the greatest and longest lasting physical morbidity, and the highest mortality rate. However, relevant issues relating to the other eating or dieting disorders are also discussed, but not obesity.

The intended audience is predominantly medical practitioners, psychiatrists, physicians, paediatricians, and general practitioners – as one of them should always be responsible for the physical health of the eating disorder patient. It is envisaged that the book will also be helpful to other health professionals involved with these patients, particularly nurses, dietitians, and also psychologists. The authors intend to produce another book on the same theme but aimed at patients, their families, and carers as well as other stakeholders such as schoolteachers and counsellors.

It is written partly as a reference textbook, partly as a manual for consultation. . . . The bibliography found at the conclusion of the book leads the reader to those papers which the authors deem to be the most noteworthy on the various issues surrounding the medical management of eating disorders.

Despite the rather authoritarian and dogmatic format, the principal authors acknowledge the limitations of their expertise. They have, between them, more than 60 years of experience in treating eating disorder patients. Whatever success they may have had is because they have stood on the shoulders of those who went before them. They trust that discussion and feedback on the book will improve their clinical practice in future.

Eating disorders are orphan conditions: everyone has opinions about them, but no discipline is willing to assume overall responsibility for their care. At one extreme, severe anorexia nervosa with cachexia, multiple nutrient deficiencies, blood and electrolyte abnormalities, and organ dysfunction is a serious physical disease with a chronic course and a high mortality rate. At the other, excessively restricted eating, obligatory exercise, and the occasional use of purging and vomiting are so common in many developed societies, particularly among young women and adolescent girls, as to be almost the norm. In between these extremes are the psychiatric illnesses of moderate anorexia nervosa, BN, atypical or eating disorder not otherwise specified, and perhaps binge eating disorder. These are mental illnesses rather than physical diseases, although they may have serious physical manifestations.

The dichotomy between mental 'illness' and physical 'disease' implies an acceptance of a dualistic view of body and mind, or soma and psyche. The authors do not wish to endorse nor refute this dualism. The opposition of dualism to physicalism had been a topic of philosophical debate long prior to Descartes' influential writings in the 14th century – and should remain so. Health care workers or clinicians are practical persons, and as such, they are concerned with the practical issues of maintaining health and combating ill health, not with esoteric issues of ultimate reality. From a clinical viewpoint both a unified and a dualistic approach has advantages. The unified view of body and mind is essential in that almost all of medicine is psychosomatic medicine; psychological factors influence physiological processes and may lead to somatic pathology; physical disease affects the mind both directly and indirectly. Thus, from a psychological perspective, we support a unified concept of body and mind. But in the real world of practice we recognise that medicine and the health professions involve two complementary approaches: one is conceived with the anatomical structure and physiological processes of the body and their distortions; the other is concerned with the contents of mind, with emotion, and with behaviour and its motivation. The diligent health care worker keeps both in mind, but is careful to distinguish in practice between that which requires physical treatment and that which requires psychological care. Perhaps nowhere else in medicine is the failure to make this distinction as disastrous as it is in respect to anorexia nervosa and its related illnesses. And, paradoxically, perhaps nowhere in medicine is it as important to run the two approaches in a complementary fashion. The therapist – or better, the team of therapists – must be physician, nurse, and dietician, as well as psychiatrist, psychologist, and mental health nurse.

The clinicians treating patients with eating disorders have a complex task. First they must identify and treat that physical disease that is caused by the dysfunctional behaviour and which is manifested in the pathology of malnutrition, chemical disturbance and organ dysfunction. Next, they must attend to the mental illness that may or may not have some physical basis (we don't know as yet). Third, they must provide help and support in respect to those aspects of these disorders that are best considered as reactions to the dilemma of controlling weight and shape in a society in which obesity has reached epidemic proportions and in which there are strong social pressures to be thinner than most people can achieve.

Good luck to those of you who chose to become involved in the management of these demanding patients. Please remember, eating disorders are legitimate illnesses. Those suffering from them deserve the same care and consideration as other sick people.

C. Laird Birmingham & Peter Beumont

Abbreviations

AE	acrodermatitis enteropathica
AN	anorexia nervosa
APA	American Psychiatric Association
ARFID	avoidant/restrictive food intake disorder
AST	aspartate transaminase
BED	binge eating disorder
BMI	body mass index (weight in kilograms divided by height in meters squared)
BN	bulimia nervosa
CPK	creatine phosphokinase
CT	computed tomography
DEXA	dual x-ray absorptiometry
DSM	*Diagnostic and Statistical Manual of Mental Disorders*
ED	eating disorder
EDNOS	eating disorder not otherwise specified
EEG	electroencephalogram
EKG	electrocardiogram
ICD	*International Classification of Diseases*
ICP	intracranial pressure
JVP	jugular venous pressure
LH	luteinising hormone
LORETA	low-resolution electromagnetic tomography of the brain
MRI	magnetic resonance imaging
OSFED	other specified feeding or eating disorder
QT interval	the time the ventricles (large chambers of the heart) take to recharge electrically
QTc	the QT interval corrected to the patient's heart rate
SMA	superior mesenteric artery
SMR	standardised mortality ratio
TE	telogen effluvium
TSH	thyroid-stimulating hormone
UFED	unspecified feeding or eating disorder
WHO	World Health Organization

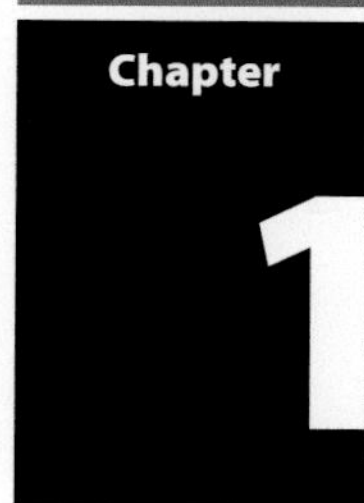

Chapter 1 Definitions and Epidemiology

Study Questions

- *A twenty-five-year-old gay man presents with frequent binging and purging. He says he wants to gain weight and become much more muscular. He appears very thin and follows a vegetarian diet.*
- *Using this case above, discuss the diagnosis you would make according to the* Diagnostic and Statistical Manual of Mental Disorders, 5th edition *(DSM-5),* International Classification of Disease, 11th edition *(ICD-11), and your own logic.*

There has been a proliferation of 'new forms' of eating disorder (ED) over the last seventy years. It started with the introduction of bulimia nervosa (BN) a Gerald Russell's seminal paper describing a case series of BN, 'an ominous variant of anorexia nervosa', in which people with a preliminary phase of anorexia lost control of eating and binge ate but used various strategies to compensate for this. BN was quickly introduced into the *DSM* and *ICD-10* classifications.

More recently, to decrease the size of the population who failed to fall into the previously described categories (ED not otherwise specified, two new diagnoses were introduced into *DSM-5*: binge ED (BED) and avoidant/restrictive food intake disorder (ARFID). The residual categories now include other specified feeding or EDs (OSFED) and feeding and EDs unspecified.

The stereotypical image of patients with EDs as thin, white middle class girls is incorrect. All sociodemographic and cultural groups are included and most are in the overweight or obese weight range. Both mental and physical health are poor and role performance is impaired.

However new variants such as diabulimia (manipulation of insulin dosing by patients with diabetes to lose weight), orthorexia (an obsession with eating foods that one considers to be healthy), and 'bigorexia' (muscle dysmorphophobia [a male ED]) are being described in the literature. Which of these have the psychosocial and physical disability sufficient to merit their classification as a disease remains to be seen.

Anorexia Nervosa

Anorexia nervosa (AN) is low in prevalence, but high in medical consequence. The most common age of onset is fifteen years (range, nine to twenty-four years). Females are diagnosed with AN ten times more often than males. During their lifetime, 0.9–2.2 per cent of women and 0.2–0.3 per cent of men are diagnosed with AN.

In addition, one-third of the cases of AN are not included in statistics, because patients have never sought treatment. The incidence of AN, the rate at which new cases

Table 1.1 Summary of the Main ED Diagnostic Criteria (adapted from the *DSM-5* criteria)

AN	Continued restriction of energy intake
	Loss of weight to below fifteen per cent of their expected weight for their age
	Intense fear of gaining weight
	Disturbed self-body image
BN	Recurrent episodes of binge eating within a short time period and of foods that are considered larger than what most people would consume during the same time period
	Lack of control of eating during binge episodes
	Recurrent compensatory behaviours, for example, self-induced vomiting
	Binge eating and compensatory behaviours occur, on average, at least once a week for three months
	Disturbed self-body image
BED	Recurrent episodes of binge eating within a short time period and of foods that are considered larger than what most people would consume during the same time period
	Binge eating episodes are associated with three or more of the following:
	Eating more rapidly than normal
	Eating until feeling uncomfortably full
	Eating large amounts of food when no physical hunger is present
	Eating alone owing to embarrassment over quantities being consumed
	Feeling disgusted or very guilty with oneself afterward
	Binge eating occurs, on average, at least once a week for three months
	No recurrent use of compensatory behaviours

occur, has not changed in the last five decades, although the incidence in adolescent girls may have increased a little.

AN has the highest mortality rate of any psychiatric condition, with a standardised mortality rate approximately ten times that of the general population. Suicide accounts for one-half the deaths; medical causes, especially arrhythmias, account for the other half. The diagnostic features of the main EDs *DSM-5* are shown in Table 1.1

Abbreviations: AN, anorexia nervosa; BED, binge eating disorder; BN, BN.

The essential feature of AN is a constant, inexplicable fear of being fat or eating, which increases with weight loss and does not change with reason.

AN is egosyntonic, which means that the patient believes their concerns about weight and shape are normal; that is, they do not think there is anything wrong with them, and they are, therefore, not interested in treatment.

Weight loss in AN is attained and sustained by insufficient food intake, usually coupled with an increase in energy expenditure caused by compulsive activity. However, one-half of cases of AN also binge eat, then vomit (binge-eating/purging subtype). Equivalents of purging that may be used in addition to, or instead of, vomiting are laxatives, enemas, suppositories, diuretics, ipecac, fasting, weight loss pills or pills to increase the metabolic rate, spitting out food, self-phlebotomy, and self-gavage.

Often patients will begin with restricting their food intake and then add exercise, which can become compulsive. Often, six months to two years later, food craving and overeating begin, presumably related to malnutrition. This drive to eat leads to binging, which then leads to purging. In one-quarter to one-half of patients with AN, the binge–purge cycle becomes chronic.

Bulimia Nervosa

Bulimia nervosa (BN) involves habitual binge eating followed by purging or a purge equivalent. The purging subtype is defined by the use of vomiting, laxatives, diuretics, or enemas. The nonpurging subtype uses other behaviours that compensate for the binge.

Patients with BN usually have a normal weight, are still active at school or work, and binge and purge covertly. However, BN is an egodystonic disorder; the patients want to be cured – although possibly not at the price of weight gain.

BN affects 1.5–2.0 per cent of women and 0.5 per cent of men. The incidence increased rapidly after the 1970s, but currently appears to be stable or possibly decreasing from a peak in the 1990s. The onset is usually in the late teenage years, later than AN.

The essential feature of BN is recurrent binge eating. A binge is defined as an episode of eating that is excessive for the context and is accompanied by a subjective sense of loss of control. The binge may be associated with reduced caloric intake, stress, a particular location (e.g., the bathroom at home), a particular time of day (e.g., at night), particular people, changes in mood, loneliness, pain, insomnia, or fatigue.

BED

BED is now in the *DSM-5*. The lifetime prevalence of BED is estimated to be 3.5 per cent among adult females and 2.0 per cent in males and the prevalence seems to be increasing. It occurs in Black as well as White ethnic groups. BED is present in about one-third of patients with obesity.

The essential feature of BED is episodes of overeating. The compulsion to overeat is often associated with the taste and quality of food, whereas in BN binges are more likely to be ritualistic and to include food that is easy to vomit afterward. There is interest in whether this might be considered as a form of food addiction. In BED, there is no extreme compensatory behaviour, like vomiting or laxative use. This behaviour is also seen in genetic forms of obesity like Prader-Willi syndrome and Kleine-Levin syndrome. There is less overinvestment in weight and shape for self-esteem than in BN.

ARFID

ARFID is often seen in younger patients. The psychopathological concern about weight and shape seen in AN is not present in ARFID, and this feature distinguishes it from AN. Different patterns of eating are encompassed in this category: avoidance of foods owing to their sensory properties (e.g., picky eating), poor appetite or limited interest in eating, abdominal or general discomfort, and fear of other negative consequences from eating.

OSFED and Unspecified Feeding or ED

This category is used for all those whose quality of life is severely affected by an ED, but who do not meet all the criteria of one of the other ED diagnoses. Despite the best efforts of the *DSM-5*, the largest number of people with EDs (approximately ten per cent) fall into these residual categories. Features of atypical AN were most common in people fitting OSFED (prevalence of three per cent). Most of those with an unspecified feeding or ED had recurrent binge eating without distress. Other examples include someone of normal weight who engages in purging such as vomiting or laxative use in the absence of binging episodes ('purging disorder').

Epidemiology of EDs

> Several recent studies have examined lifetime prevalence rates using *DSM-5* criteria and the prevalence of AN ranges from 0.8–3.6 per cent, BN from 0.28–2.10 per cent, and BED from 0.4–1.9 per cent. There has only one study that has reported the incidence of cases of EDs. The latest report used *DSM-IV* criteria and found incident rates per 100,000 of 7.9 per cent for AN, 11.8 per cent for BN, and 17.1 per cent for ED not otherwise specified presenting to primary care in the UK.

Implications for Health Care Professionals

- ED not otherwise specified has been dropped from the *DSM-5*. The new diagnostic categories are BED, ARFID, OSFED, and unspecified feeding or ED.

Patient Explanation

- The new categorisation of EDs is similar to changing the name of tidal waves to tsunamis. It does not change the importance of your ED. However, it might change whether the treatment of your ED is covered by insurance as well the current 'standard' therapy that you may be offered.

Section 2 Cause

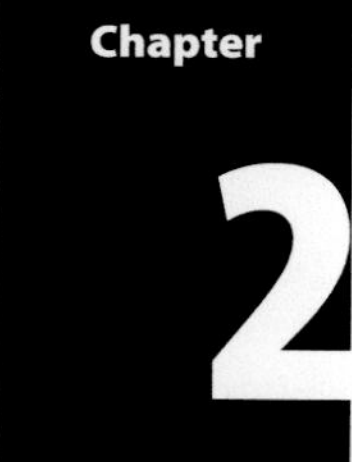

Chapter 2 Causal and Maintaining Factors

Study Questions

- *Are eating disorders caused by pressure from the media to conform to ideals of weight and shape?*
- *Is the prevalence of anorexia nervosa and bulimia nervosa the same around the world? Give some hypotheses to explain any differences.*
- *Will someone who has 'recovered' from anorexia nervosa continue to have food, weight, and shape preoccupation? For how long? How about bulimia nervosa? Do those who suffer from obesity have increased weight and shape concerns?*

The causal models of eating disorders (EDs) should explain the differential epidemiology between anorexia nervosa (AN) and binge EDs (BEDs). Why has the prevalence of AN remained low over its long history, in contrast with the exponential increase of BEDs, which are common problems, particularly in women born in the latter half of the twentieth century? Why is binge eating more common in urban environments?

It is probable that the cultural factors that account for the rapid increase in the prevalence of obesity within this timeframe also contribute to the risk of bulimia nervosa (BN) and BEDs. Cultural factors may contribute to the maintenance of all forms of EDs, making them impermeable to therapy.

For those interested in examining risk factors in more depth, the primary sources are contained in a systematic review by Jacobi and colleagues.

Cultural Factors

Western culture, which has fostered the idealisation of thinness and market-driven self-discontent, promotes the possibility of a self makeover, given the expenditure of enough resources. The tension between fear of food and its consequences, in the context of a market that promotes highly palatable foods and foods that have been technologically tweaked to be appealing, promotes anxiety and EDs. Peers and family members may reinforce cultural body ideals through fat talk – namely, weight stigma and teasing. Loss of the social connectivity provided by sharing meals, combined with easy access to anonymously obtained food in our permissive urban environment, sets the scene for binge eating.

Biological Risk Factors

Genetics

EDs often run in families. The risk is increased ten-fold. The heritability estimates from twin and family studies for both AN and BN are about sixty per cent. Several family-based linkage studies have identified loci for AN, BN, or associated behavioural traits. Extremely large populations are needed to robustly identify candidate genes. Work is in progress to build this information for EDs. It is probable that a number of genes, each of which has a small effect, contributes to an increase in risk.

The results so far suggest that there are many overlaps between the profile of genes associated with AN and other psychiatric disorders, such as obsessive–compulsive disorder and schizophrenia. Interestingly, there are also overlaps with genes associated with growth and metabolism (e.g., a negative correlation with body mass index and a positive correlation with insulin sensitivity). In addition, the risks associated with these genes may only be expressed in the presence of other specific risk factor(s), like weight loss. Thus, the genetics of EDs can be considered a work in progress.

Perinatal Risk Factors

People who develop EDs are more likely to have a history of obstetric complications, such as prematurity, small-for-dates, and cephalohematoma. Adverse perinatal factors such as higher levels of maternal stress are also more likely. The presence of these factors may increase the risk of EDs because they are associated with anomalies in placental functioning, impacting brain development and hypothalamic–pituitary–adrenal dysfunction. It is possible that nutritional–epigenetic mechanisms may account for the impact on metabolism and/or stress responsivity.

Neurophysiological Vulnerabilities

Between the genotype and the clinical phenotypes that fluctuate in response to environmental circumstances are underlying risk components called endophenotypes. The endophenotypes are the measurable metabolic, electrophysiological, endocrinological, anatomical, or cognitive/psychological/neuropsychological risk factors. Endophenotypes are often evaluated using data regarding developmental and personality disorders. This process has led to the examination of endophenotypes associated with autistic spectrum disorders and obsessive–compulsive traits, particularly for AN and for endophenotypes relating to attention deficit hyperactivity disorder and the emotionally unstable, borderline type of personality for BEDs.

AN Endophenotypes

People with EDs (particularly at the AN end of the spectrum) share similar information processing styles with people on the autistic spectrum conditions and with obsessive–compulsive disorder in that they have weak set shifting (a rigid, perseverative style) and weak central coherence (a tendency to focus on detail and a relative weakness in integrating into a global perspective). These cognitive biases are associated with behavioural traits such as inflexibility, sensitivity to error, and perfectionism.

Biology Meets the Environment

Environmental triggers causing stress, loss of weight, or a change in meal content or patterning can exaggerate or activate the endophenotypic traits and perpetuate the problem. Weight loss itself increases rigidity, compulsivity, and a narrow focus, particularly if these traits are dormant in the individual. These traits stimulate rule-driven behaviours relating to the intake and expenditure of calories. The focus on detail and habitual patterns allow a feed-forward pattern to develop. The individual has difficulty stepping back to see the bigger picture and how their overall quality of life is destroyed.

Binge Eating Endophenotypes

BEDs are associated with traits of disinhibition and heightened reward sensitivity. The reward system is a key part of the central regulation of appetite. Animal studies suggest that there are both innate and acquired differences in reward systems that impact on eating behaviour. There is also an association between attention deficit hyperactivity disorder and a shared endophenotype of impulsivity and problems with attention.

Innate Anomalies in Reward Sensitivity

Between and within animal species, there are innate variations in reward sensitivity to food. An increased sensitivity to food reward may explain the co-segregation of obesity, the bulimic disorders, and the overeating style in childhood, seen in developmental studies.

Acquired Anomalies in Reward Sensitivity

Animal models of binge eating have been developed that involve an increased sensitisation of reward systems. The conditions that lead to a pattern of binge eating in laboratory animals involve experimental manipulation of the environment, such as a period of starvation, artificial diversion of food from the stomach, stress, and intermittent access to highly palatable food. These animal models also show an increased appetite for addictive substances. The underlying mechanisms seem to involve physiological changes in the reward systems of the brain, with alterations in dopamine, opiate, and endocannabinoid systems.

The environmental contingencies that produce binge eating in animals are some of the key environmental factors and behaviours that are associated with the changes in the epidemiology of EDs. If we generalise the findings of animal research to humans, chaotic dieting, vomiting, and stress result in acquired changes to the reward system, which may exaggerate and perpetuate the disruption of appetite by producing addictive changes in the brain. This mechanism may underpin the transition from AN to BN, and explain why food craving and binge eating are common sequelae of a period of restricting AN. The neurotic fear that the anorexic must control and subjugate her appetite or it will rise up and overwhelm her can become a reality by this mechanism.

A General Causal Model for EDs

A model explaining these causal and maintaining factors for EDs is shown in Figure 2.1. This diagram illustrates the genetic, environmental, and developmental factors that can interact, over the life trajectory, to increase the risk of developing an ED. The top box illustrates the range of clinical phenotypes with the various forms of ED ranging from restricting AN to obesity.

The various networks that may have anomalous functionality because of genetic variation (stress, reward, and appetite systems) are shown in the bottom box. Between these two boxes are the endophenotypes. In the diagram, we have restricted these endophenotypes to some of the cognitive and rewards systems; however, it is probable that further endophenotypes will be discovered, for example, an emotional endophenotype

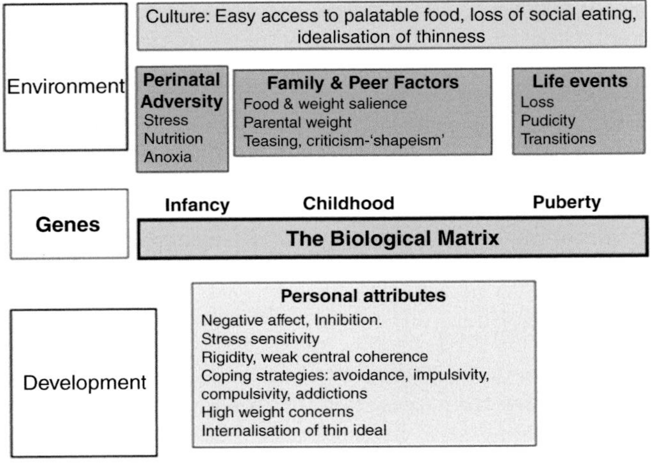

Figure 2.1 Risk factors within the cultural, environmental, genetic, and psychological domains that contribute to the development of eating disorders over the life course.

may explain the increase in fear sensitivity. Anomalies in social cognition may explain some of the social alienation described by people with AN. The environment can interact with these traits, exaggerating them, contributing to a positive feedback trap. Thus, starvation and stress increase rigidity and a tendency to tunnel vision. In conjunction with traits of disinhibition, starvation and stress can lead to intermittent ingestion of highly palatable foods, which can produce reward sensitisation, an addictive response to food and other substances.

The Factors That Maintain EDs

In the section on A General Causal Model for EDs, we have described how biological elements can be activated by the environment and act as maintaining factors. By definition, maintaining factors are those variables that predict symptom persistence over time among initially symptomatic individuals. Identifying maintaining factors is important because their successful treatment is often necessary for recovery.

AN

A four-factor model of maintenance has been developed for AN. This includes two dispositions that precede the onset:

(1) Compulsive traits, rigidity, and perfectionism; and

(2) High anxiety and avoidance.

The impact of starvation on the cognitive endophenotype that exaggerates compulsivity and perfectionist traits was discussed in the section, The Factors That Maintain EDs. There are other consequences of severe starvation that have to do with its meaning for the individual. These include:

(3) The reactions, of those who are close, with features of high expressed emotion (overprotection and criticism) and behaviours that inadvertently enable the anorexic behaviours; and

(4) Biological and psychological changes that are perceived as positive by the individual.

The Evolution of ED Symptoms

The pattern of secondary consequences evolves over time. The early phase is common to all forms of ED; however, the pathways diverge depending on whether dietary rules producing marked weight loss continue or whether homeostatic forces, which drive eating to restore body weight, prevail.

The Early Phase of an ED

In the early phase, peers and family may applaud the individual with an ED for her application to food and exercise rules, which give the impression of following a healthy lifestyle. This phase is shared by all forms of EDs. Usually, there is, in addition, a more concentrated application to academic work with less interest in social activities, and this behaviour is seen as commendable. For the individual herself, the success and sense of mastery that the application to the detail of dietary rules has on her goals is rewarding.

The Later Phase: Visible Emaciation in AN

The later phase of those with the traits that allow the unremitting weight loss to continue tipping them into AN, a variety of secondary gains can occur. The overt display of starvation pain causes others who are close to them to react. Family members draw idiosyncratic meanings from the ED behaviours. The emotional reactions of family members can oscillate from anger and frustration, to care and concern, or avoidance. Some of these reactions to the ED behaviours can inadvertently be rewarding. Family members may give attention or credence to the ED voice, or they may remove negative consequences that arise from the ED behaviour. The family may accept that EDs symptoms dominate the household: becoming subservient to ED food rules (where, why, how, when, and with whom, etc.), safety behaviours (exercise, vomiting, body checking, fasting, or cutting back), and obsessive–compulsive behaviours (reassurance seeking, counting, checking, and control). The individual with an ED controls those around him or her by explicit or implicit emotional blackmail. For example, if ED rules are disobeyed, then the patient threatens to not eat at all, or to harm herself or himself, or act destructively in other ways. Thus, the overt communication of distress of AN may bully the family so that they submit to ED rules and accommodate to the illness.

The respect and care given to those in the sick role can make the person with an ED special. The individual with an ED may control, compete, compare, or calibrate herself or himself with other family members (often siblings) in terms of what and how much to eat or exercise. Again, this behaviour is tolerated in an effort to keep the peace, and because there is fear about resisting.

Pro Starvation Beliefs

In addition to the positive interpersonal consequences that result from the behaviour, there can be secondary physical and psychological consequences that are reinforcing for the individual. For example, the emotional numbing that follows from starvation can aid the avoidance of painful emotions. An avoidant response to emotional arousal and insecure attachments are common predisposing traits in AN. We have discussed in Biology Meets the Environment how the exaggeration of rigidity and focus on detail can have positive benefits in following dietary rules and attaining goals that become reinforcing. The poor concentration and decision making that are associated with starvation impact the capacity to show mature reflective functioning and effective problem-solving capacities. This means that the capacity to assimilate treatment and the concerns of responsible others is impaired.

Similarly, physical consequences may be perpetuating. Physical debility and poor concentration can heighten the patient's sense of vulnerability and personal inadequacy. This need to bolster a frail sense of self drives them to continue a pattern of behaviour that gives them a sense of mastery. Secondary effects on gastrointestinal function, such as slowed gastric emptying and constipation, may contribute to the discomfort and bloating that are the common complaints of individuals when they start to eat. In some cases, the decrease in the secretion of sex hormones is welcomed. It may provide relief from the challenges of menstruation and from sexual demands.

The Later Phase: The Evolution of Craving and the Development of Binge Eating

In those patients with traits of disinhibition and heightened reward sensitivity, the craving to eat will become intense. The hormones released or suppressed by starvation alter the sensitivity of the reward centre of the brain (e.g., low leptin levels increase the sensitivity to reward). Thus, the drive to eat can become irresistible. Foods that are easily accessible and highly palatable are more desired. After the initial hurried pleasure from eating, there is a negative rebound of mood. The individual becomes concerned at her lack of satiation to food and is concerned that her appetite will have no boundaries, that unless she exerts stringent controls she will expand to be an elephant. The experience of self-control and failure will lead her to make reparation and then to make a fresh start, with even more stringent dietary rules. BEDs are usually conducted in secret. The individual is all too aware of the false persona that she exhibits to the world. She may keep people at a distance for fear that they see the dark side of her life. The resources and chaos that binge eating produce in the kitchen and bathroom can cause difficulties for people sharing the facilities. Guilt and disgust lowers self-esteem further and there are renewed attempts to be good.

Developing a Formulation

The diagnostic systems of classification remain in a state of flux. Furthermore, it is possible that a similar diagnostic presentation can result from a different underlying mechanism. This is the basic premise of personalised/precision psychiatry. The

Table 2.1 The three facets of a formulation predisposing, precipitating, and perpetuating factors

Predisposing	Genetics: polygenic correlation with obsessive–compulsive disorder, schizophrenia, metabolic factors Environmental stress: prenatal onwards Temperament: autism spectrum disorder, attention deficit hyperactivity disorder, obsessive–compulsive personality disorder, anxiety, shyness
Precipitating	Specific triggers: fat talk, weight stigma, type of food General triggers: loss, social exclusion/shame
Perpetuating	Secondary gains: physical, psychological, social, behavioural

formulation is a traditional clinical tool that exemplifies a personalised approach. It includes the risk factors that may have predisposed to, or precipitated, or perpetuated (the three *P*s) the individual's ED. These can be categorised into physical, psychological, and social factors. A shared formulation is an important first step in the process of engagement. Some of the typical risk factors for the various forms of ED are shown in Table 2.1. In many forms of therapy, the formulation is personalised and used to target treatment. The perpetuating factors are a particular focus.

Obtaining the History and Physical Examination

Study Questions

- *Design a history and investigation protocol in the style of a 'fill in the blank' form that you could use in your practice.*
- *What complications of an eating disorder are irreversible?*
- *Self-injurious behaviour is common in patients with eating disorders. Can self-injurious behaviour be diagnosed on physical examination?*
- *Which physical signs of eating disorders are specific to anorexia nervosa? To bulimia nervosa?*

Obtaining the History

Leave your office to meet the patient where they are waiting. This action provides an opportunity to observe their behaviour with those who have accompanied them. Take note of their affect, strength, steadiness, movement, and gait. Introduce yourself to the family and friends who have accompanied the patient. Their deportment, anxiety, and apparent closeness to the patient is highly relevant. Consider the implication of a number of family members who accompany the patient and who ask for and take your instructions versus a dominant parent who does not allow their child to speak and forces their way into the interview. It is important to have some of the interview with the patient themselves. Ask the parent whether a colleague or assistant could join you, if the parent does not want to leave the child alone with you.

Certain elements of the history, such as those related to abuse or sexual issues, are best left to a subsequent interview when rapport has been developed. Table 3.1 presents a schema for history recording.

The Physical Examination

Have the patient change privately, keep their underwear on, and wear the gown with the opening to the back. If the patient is hesitant about being examined, ask why. Do not start or even undertake the physical examination unless you are certain the patient is totally aware of and agrees to the extent of the examination before starting. If they are not, do a limited examination or have a parent, friend, or one of your colleagues present if that reassures the patient.

Examining a fully dressed patient will prevent observation of the degree of emaciation, signs of self-injurious behaviour, heart sounds and murmur, surgical scars, sacral oedema, hardening stool, and other physical signs. A cursory examination reinforces the

Table 3.1 Obtaining the medical history of patients with eating disorders

Identifying information

Name

Date of birth

Address

Phone: Work Home Mobile

Permission to contact: to protect confidentiality, obtain the specifics of where you may contact the patient (who, where, how?)

Referral source

Date and time of examination

History of present illness

Was history also obtained from collateral sources?

Weight

Pregnancy and birth

Was the mother (foetus) overnourished or undernourished during the pregnancy?

Weight at birth, from five to ten years of age, and during the teens. How did it vary over time?

Adult weight

Maximum weight

Usual weight

Preferred weight

Lowest weight

Desire for weight change

Desired weight

Healthiest weight

Periods of weight loss and gain; include how, why, and any lasting effect

Attitudes towards shape and size

Feelings about size and shape

Weight: There is usually a difference between the weight the patient believes would be medically acceptable and that which she desires.

Eating behaviour

Eating: average day at present

Breakfast Snack Lunch Snack Dinner Snack

List of the foods that they can eat and keep down

List of the foods that they will not eat

Food allergies/intolerances: which food and what happens?

Vegetarian? Vegan? When did this begin?

Intolerance to certain foods (e.g., lactose)

Food preferences

Religious and cultural beliefs about foods

Table 3.1 *(cont.)*

Time course of their beliefs about food

Do they have beliefs about food composition?

Adaptive behaviours

Exercise

Current pattern of exercise

Types of exercising (aerobic/anaerobic)

Most extreme exercise

Duration of exercise in 24 hours

Is exercise obligatory?

Effects of missing a day of exercise

Debit (e.g., what food would they not eat?)

Do they have non-exercise activity (fidgeting, standing, constantly moving, chewing, discomfort if they have to remain still)?

Purging

How long after binge?

Do they fluid load (to make vomiting easier)?

How (e.g., fingers, toothbrush, contract abdomen)?

Number of times they vomit during each episode of purging.

Is blood vomited? How often? How much?

Other methods of purging (what, how much, when?)

Laxatives, enemas, suppositories

Diuretics, ipecac, herbal or over-the-counter weight loss remedies

Fasting, exercise, misuse of insulin, self-phlebotomy, self-gavage

Suck and spit, ruminative behaviour

Purging behaviours: take a history of all the purging behaviours that have been used, not just at present. Taking a very detailed history of purging usually decreases the patient's anxiety by revealing the secret and understanding that these behaviours are common.

Binge eating

First binged When? Where? Why?

Usual binge What? Times the amount of a normal meal?

Ever binge with others?

Feelings during binge

Length of binge Why does the binge stop? How do they feel during and after the binge?

Physical symptoms

Head and neck

Hair loss, new growth

Vision: Night vision: does their vision go out of focus after reading for fifteen to thirty minutes?

Table 3.1 *(cont.)*

Skin: Dry Bruising Rash

Cardiovascular/respiratory

Shortness of breath, orthopnoea, paroxysmal nocturnal dyspnoea, exercise tolerance

Palpitations sudden onset/finish frequency duration

Change recently? Related to binge and purge? Rapid or slow rate?

Regular or irregular rhythm? Do they feel dizzy or faint during the palpitations?

Do they feel hot and sweaty when they should feel cold and vice versa?

Does their heart rate speed up for hours or go slow for hours unrelated to activity?

Chest pain: Where? Precipitating factors, radiation

Associated symptoms: description (knife, ache, burning, heaviness, etc.)

Duration? Relieving factors?

Autonomic dysfunction is suggested by marked variation in heart rate, perspiration or bowel or bladder function with no apparent cause. This may indicate an increased risk of arrhythmia and sudden death.

Sexual and reproductive/menstrual history

Frequency: periodicity, flow, amenorrhoea

Oral contraceptives, anovulation, pregnancy, mothering

Any concerns about the effect of the eating disorder on fertility, pregnancy and health of children?

Urinary

Incontinence, stress incontinence

Nocturia, urinary frequency and volume

Is there intermittent rectal prolapse that effects urination?

Musculoskeletal

Strength (decreased ability to exercise?) Weakness (where?)

Cramps (where, when?) numbness, pain

(describe)

Neurological

Handed (right or left)

Dizziness (describe)

Any change in concentration, memory (short term and long term), judgment, insight, maths skills

Psychosocial

How much time do they spend thinking about weight, shape, eating concerns?

Can they eat in front of others? Who?

What specific effect has the eating disorder had on their life?

Change in mood: Does their mood swing? Depression, suicidal ideation

Table 3.1 *(cont.)*

Have they had any impulse to steal food or other things?
Have they hurt themselves?
Past medical history
Personal history
Allergies, including medication and possible food allergies or intolerances. When, what happened, what treatment was given?
Medication history: what, how much, can they afford them, do they purge them, how could they keep them down?
What over-the-counter medications do they take (or have taken)? Illicit drugs used? Have they been habituated or addicted to substances?
Cigarettes (How many? How long?)
Alcohol: wine, beer, hard liquor? How much?
Binge drinking? Do they ever use alcohol to manage their feelings or behaviour?
Smoking can be an anorexic behaviour (10 calories of energy are burned per cigarette)
Family history
History of eating disorders, substance abuse, mental disease, high or low weight, extreme exercise or abnormal eating
Functional inquiry

patient's feeling of worthlessness – why would you examine them fully when nothing is wrong with them? It is preferable to perform the physical examination on females in the presence of a female trusted by the patient or a female staff person.

Do not perform a rectal, pelvic, or breast examination as part of an eating disorder assessment examination. If the history or physical exam suggest they are indicated, have the patient ask their family physician to perform them.

A physical examination should be performed when the patient first presents for assessment and repeated subsequently depending on symptoms and weight gain. Table 3.2 presents an outline of the physical examination. Figure 3.1 shows a mnemonic of physical signs seen in eating disorders.

Repeat the physical examination if there are new or changing signs of symptoms, such as a rapid increase or decrease in weight, loss of consciousness, confusion, dizziness, palpitations, weakness, pain, fever, muscle cramps or spasms, self-injurious behaviour, or a decrease in serum sodium, potassium, magnesium, or phosphorus.

In addition, frequent physical examination is indicated if the patient has a history of underreporting or they have self-injurious behaviour. Symptoms may not be reported owing to embarrassment, low self-esteem, belief that no one cares, lack of enough energy to report owing to depression or severe malnutrition, experience with uncaring health care professionals, belief their concerns will be interpreted as criticism, belief it will be taken as proof they have been lying or underreported previously, or fear of treatment or certification that might result. For example, the patient will not report self-injurious behaviour if they have been told they will be discharged from treatment – unless they want to be discharged from treatment.

Photographs 1 through 12 illustrate common or important physical findings (see Plate section between pages 18 and 19).

Table 3.2 The physical examination

Element	Comments
General inspection	Clothing: bulky clothing, may be worn to hide weight loss, or blatant underdressing to display emaciation or for cold exposure.
Vital signs Temperature (ear/mouth/axillary/other) Blood pressure (appropriate cuff size) Right, left Sitting Standing Lying Respiratory rate	Always measure both the blood pressure and the heart rate. Take blood pressure and heart rate in at least one arm with the patient lying and standing. If there is decrease of more than 10 mm Hg in diastolic blood pressure or ten beats per minute increase in heart rate, retake the blood pressure and heart rate every fifteen seconds until stable.
Head and neck Hair (alopecia) Eyes (lateral nystagmus) Teeth (erosion) Gums (recession, friable) Parotid hypertrophy Submandibular gland hypertrophy Thyroid (normal, enlarged, nodule)	The most common cause of alopecia is hair loss owing to malnutrition. It is a generalised loss of scalp hair with no sign of inflammation or abnormality of the hair follicle. The most common gaze abnormality of Wernicke's encephalopathy is lateral nystagmus (on lateral gaze the eye moves rapidly back and forth). With vomiting the parotid and submandibular glands are swollen bilaterally. This symptom can also occur with malnutrition alone, although the swelling is usually less marked. The glands are not swollen on one side of the body only.
Cardiorespiratory Irregular rhythm Jugular venous pressure Chest Heart sounds (midsystolic clicks/murmur)	A sinus arrhythmia, in which the heart rate increases immediately after inspiration, is common and normal in those under twenty years of age. Midsystolic clicks of mitral valve prolapse are heard at the left lower sternal border to the apex and are increased by doing the Valsalva manoeuvre while standing.
Abdominal Abdomen (stool/liver/spleen/mass)	An abdominal mass that can be indented is always stool.
Skin Skin (dryness, peeling of skin of hands and feet) Hypercarotenaemia	Acrocyanosis describes extremities that are constantly a blue colour. This is usually due to slow movement of blood. This allows for greater extraction of oxygen from the blood, leading to desaturation of the blood and resulting in cyanosis. Raynaud's phenomenon is no more common in AN than in those without AN.

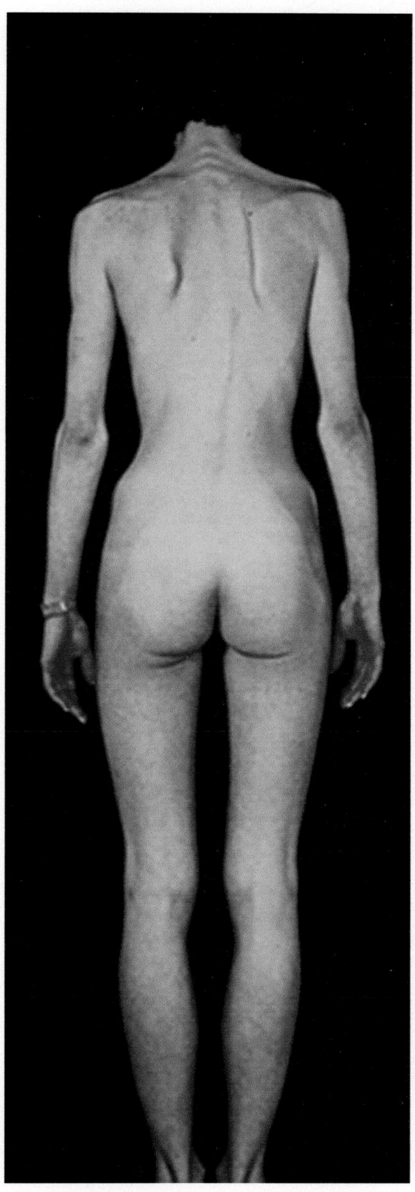

Photograph 1: Wasting. Generalized muscle wasting is apparent in addition to markedly reduced subcutaneous fat. Muscle wasting is often most evident by the loss of the convexity of the temporal muscles, the increased prominence of the scapulae and the ribs, the obvious lower rib margin, the increased prominence of the anterior superior iliac spine, and the wasting of the gluteal muscles. However, muscles that were large before weight loss (thigh muscles in bicyclists) may not appear wasted, even with marked reduction in size.

Photograph 2: Pitting oedema. Pitting oedema means that a pit or indentation will be caused by the application of localized pressure on the surface of the body. The pit is due to excess water in the tissues – just like the footprints that are formed when you walk in mud. The excess fluid in the tissues accumulates if movement of fluid into the blood is reduced due to inadequate serum protein, if there is increased pressure pushing it out of the blood as in heart failure, or if the body accumulates too much fluid to handle, as in kidney failure or during the refeeding process. Edema is usually dependent, where gravity has caused the excess water to collect. Just like mud forms where the water gathers in the lower parts of a path. So, test for it in the ankles at the end of the day or over the sacrum first thing in the morning. During sleep it accumulates in the middle of the body, as shown in this picture. In children and adolescents who often sleep face down, edema may be most evident on the face in the morning.

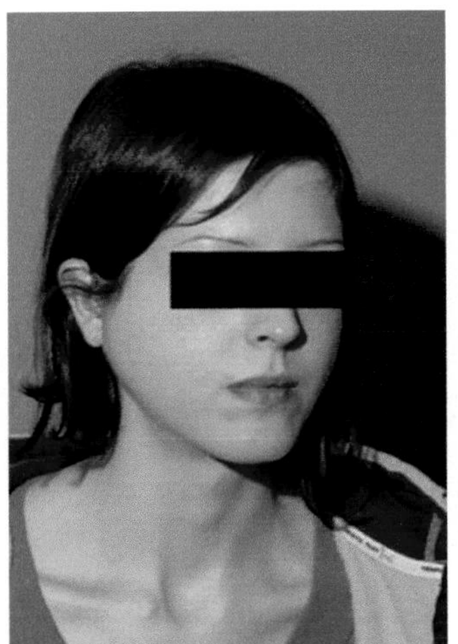

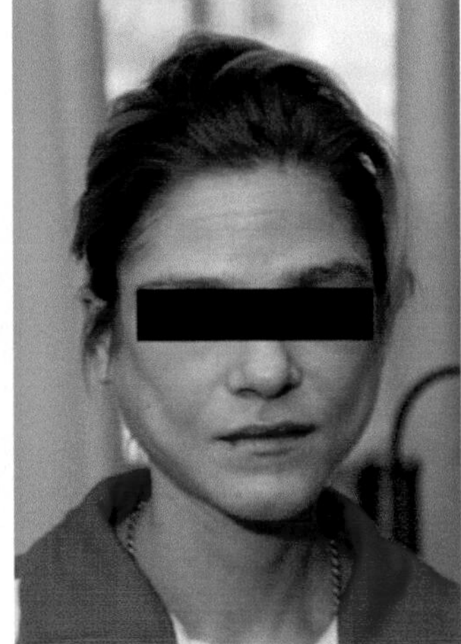

Photograph 3 & 4: Parotid hypertrophy. The parotid gland in healthy people is about the size of a small oyster. It lies just in front of the ear and above the line of the jaw. If there is enlargement of the parotid gland, called parotid hypertrophy, the face appears wider, and the ears may stick out a little. Sometimes there is a clear line demarcating the edge of the parotid – sometimes not. When you palpate the parotid and find it enlarged it clearly makes the face appear wider. I always let the patient know that their face is wider because of parotid hypertrophy because it is an incentive to recover. Protein-calorie malnutrition without vomiting often causes mild parotid hypertrophy. Thus there can have mild parotid hypertrophy in anorexia nervosa restricting subtype. Parotid hypertrophy is more pronounced with vomiting. When vomiting increases in frequency the parotid usually rapidly enlarges and becomes uncomfortable and tender to the touch.

Stensen's duct, which drains the salivary fluid from the parotid gland into the mouth, may become more prominent with purging. It appears as a little prominence with a cavity in the middle, inside the mouth just above the second lower molar bilaterally. The submandibular glands, which lie just below the jaw near the corner of the mouth, enlarge in the same way that the parotid gland does. Occasionally a patient will report enlarged lymph nodes, mistaking the enlarged submandibular glands for lymph nodes.

The parotid gland may also be enlarged in mumps, other viral infections, acute suppurative parotitis, stone blocking the duct, alcoholism, Sjogren's syndrome, or tumour. If one parotid enlarges quickly and is very tender in eating disorder patient, acute suppurative parotitis should be considered.

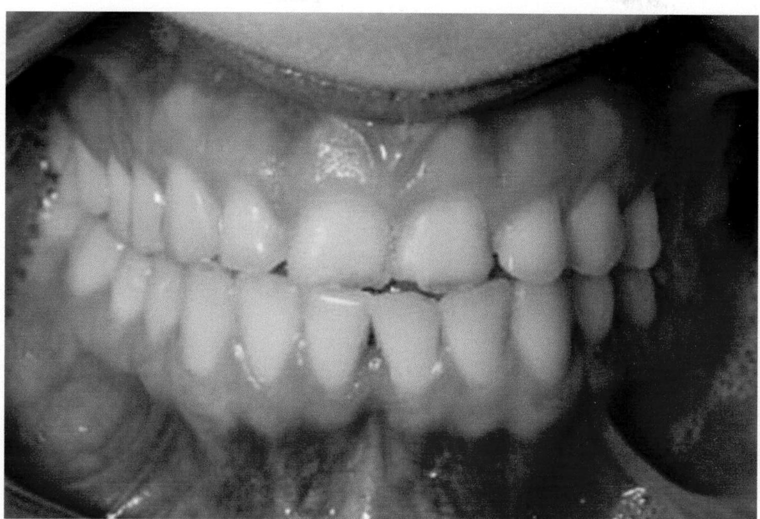

Photograph 5: Teeth and gums. The teeth in this photograph are extremely thin and very sensitive to hot or cold food or fluid. This patient will likely have dentures in her early 30s. Vomiting food, acid, or bile erodes the teeth. The gums become friable and recede. Inflammation at the corners of the mouth may be due to riboflavin deficiency (angular stomatitis). Loss of the velvety coating of the tongue, most evident by loss of the fungiform papillae at the back of the tongue (depapillation), can result from a deficiency of vitamin B_{12}, folate, or less commonly iron. Bleeding of friable gums may be a sign of scurvy.

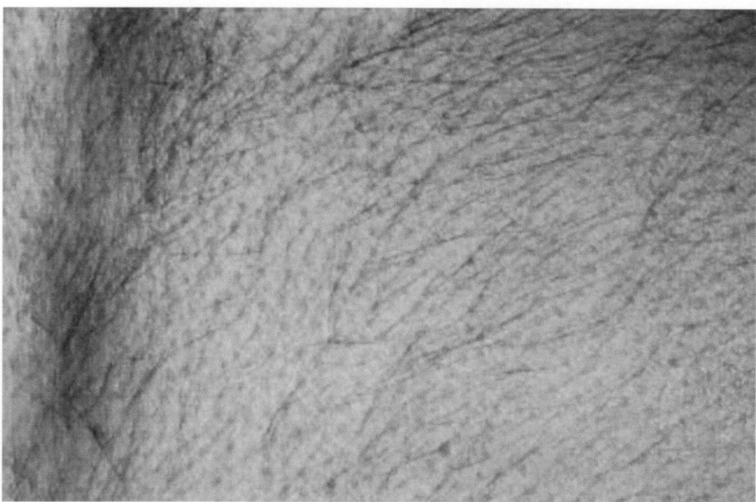

Photograph 6: Lanugo hair. This fine hair is a sign of severe malnutrition in anorexia nervosa, it looks like the fine hair seen on newborns. Lanugo hair is most easily appreciated on the abdomen or back. The pigmentation of lanugo hair is the same as the pigmentation of the patient's normal hair. Lanugo hair disappears with recovery.

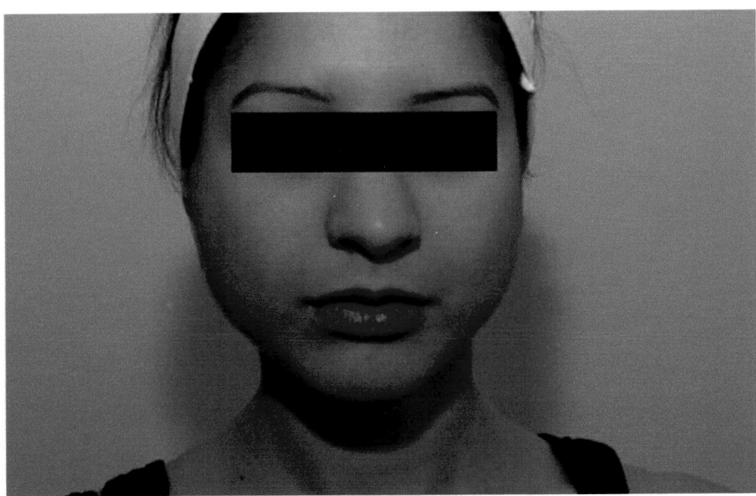

Photograph 7: Lanugo hair on the face seen as 'fuzzy' hair. This patient has bilateral parotid hypertrophy.

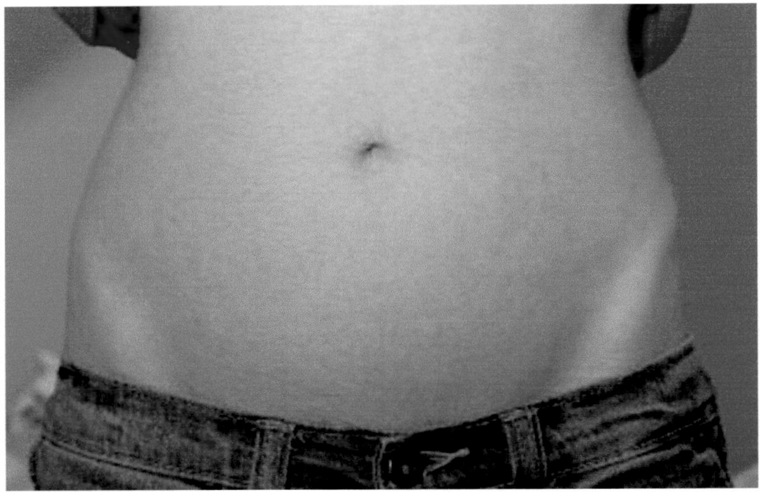

Photograph 8: In this picture, lanugo hair is present on the lower abdomen. The patient has a fair complexion, so the lanugo hair is fair in colour too. This makes it more difficult to appreciate. However, when looking from the side the density of these fine hairs are obvious.

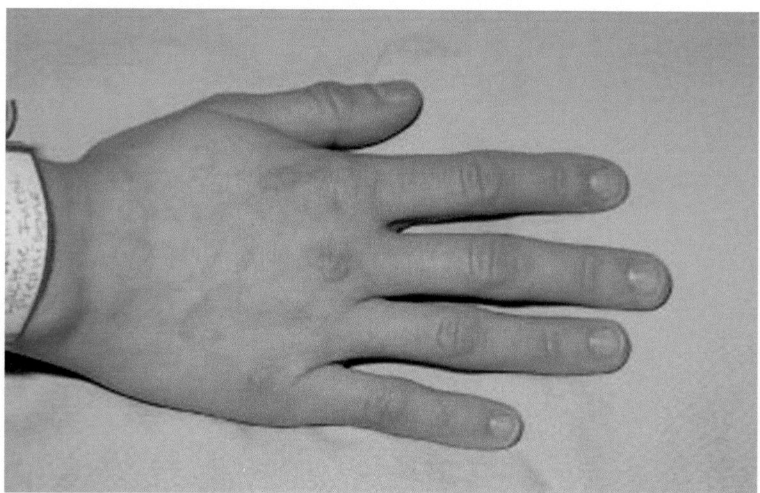

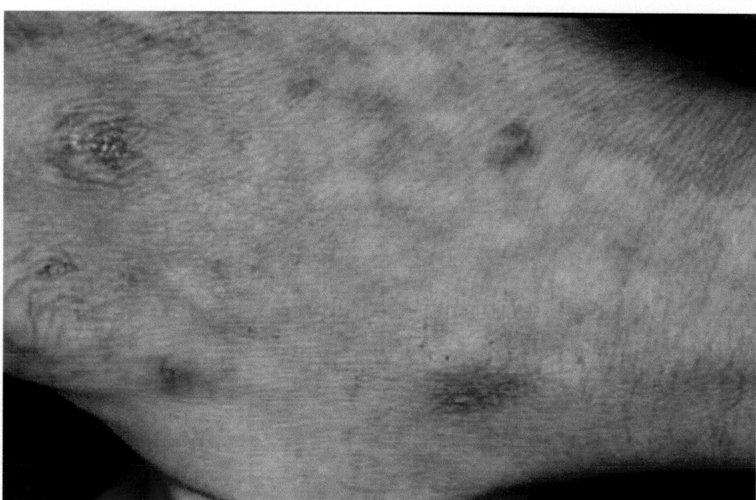

Photograph 9 & 10: Russell's sign is the scarring on the back of the hand caused by repeatedly inducing vomiting by pushing the hand against the teeth. Russell's sign is seen less frequently because more patients over the past three decades quickly learn to induce vomiting at will or by pressing on their abdomen. The scars do not disappear. Russell's sign is named after Professor Gerald Russell who first described it. These two photographs demonstrate some of the range in pigmentation of this scarring.

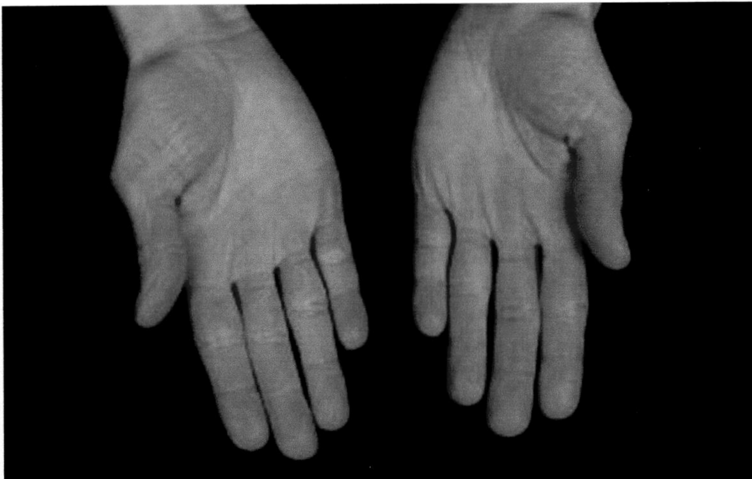

Photograph 11: Acrocyanosis. The blue/purple hue of the skin of the hands and feet is frequent, obvious, but usually overlooked. Acrocyanosis is caused by reduced blood flow to the extremities due to deoxygenated haemoglobin due to vasoconstriction that results from cold stress and volume depletion. It disappears early in treatment.

Often patients are misdiagnosed with Raynaud's disease. Raynaud's is diagnosed when there is repeated colour change of hands or other parts of the body, between at least two of white, red, and purple. Raynaud's may be associated with other diseases such as collagen vascular disease.

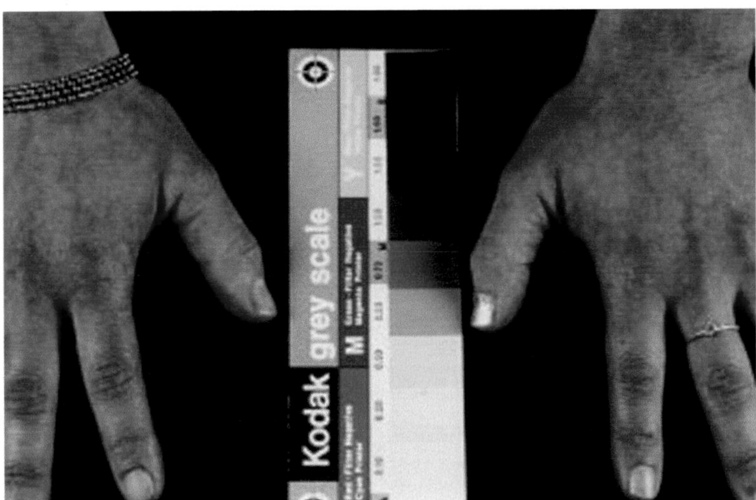

Photograph 12: Hypercarotenaemia is present when the patient's body is yellow, but their eyes remain white. In contrast, in jaundice both the body and eyes are yellow. Comparing your hands to those of the patient is often the best way to check for yellow skin. Be careful, both hands may appear yellow if the light is dim or something in the environment (for example, medical curtains) is yellow. Carotene bound to elastin in the tissues causes no symptoms, whereas jaundice may be associated with pruritis. The patient with hypercarotenaemia should have yellow skin, white sclera, and no itch.

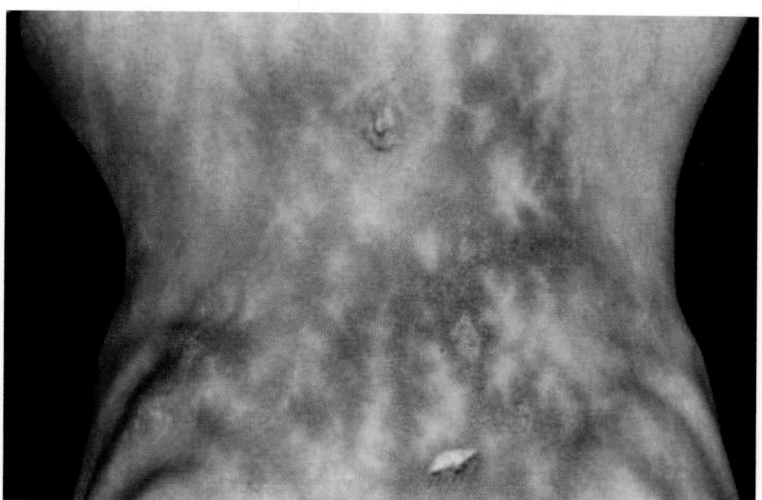

Photograph 13: Erythema ab igne. This rash is a poorly circumscribed darkening area of the skin to which the patient has habitually applied heat. It is without symptoms and does not vary in location from day to day. It is usually present over the abdomen or lower back. The hyperpigmentation may be permanent but may decrease if the patient stops heating that area of skin. The patient learns that heat makes them feel better by warming them and reducing anxiety.

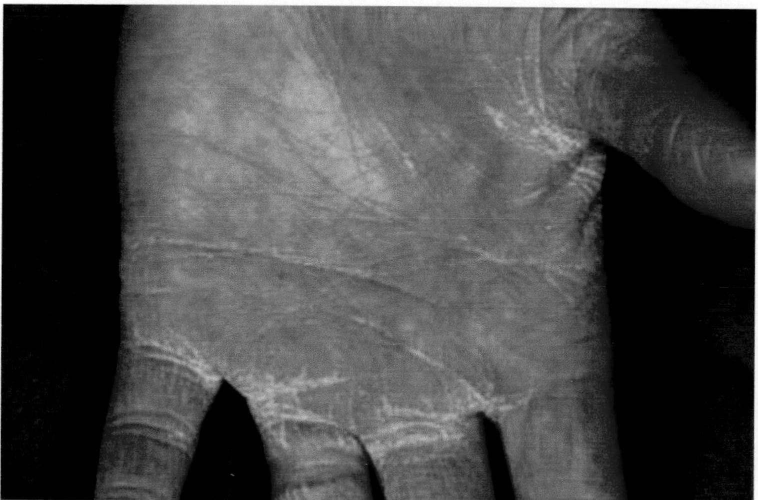

Photograph 14: Acrodermatitis. Acrodermatitis is the very dry and somewhat scaly skin on the palms and soles caused by zinc deficiency. Skin is often dry and scaly in eating disorders due to excessive washing, but not as markedly as in acrodermatitis. Zinc deficiency also causes an abnormal taste sensation (dysgeusia), alters eating behaviour, decreases immunity, and results in poor or incomplete healing of skin abrasions.

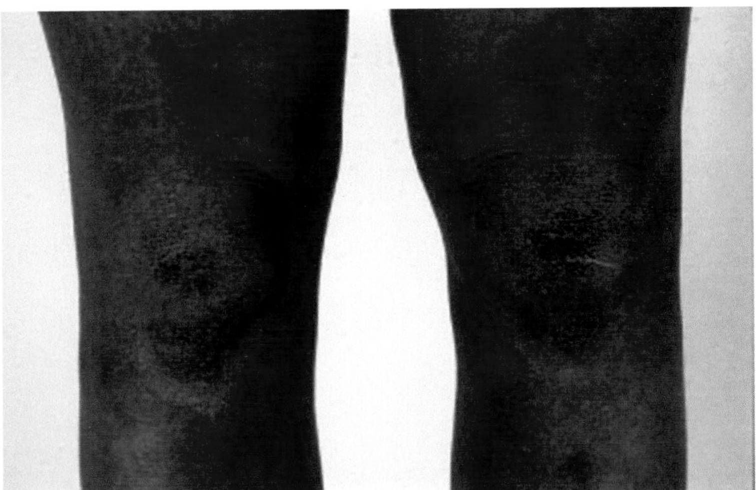

Photograph 15: Pellagra. A dark flaky rash located over the front of the lower extremities should raise the suspicion of pellagra.

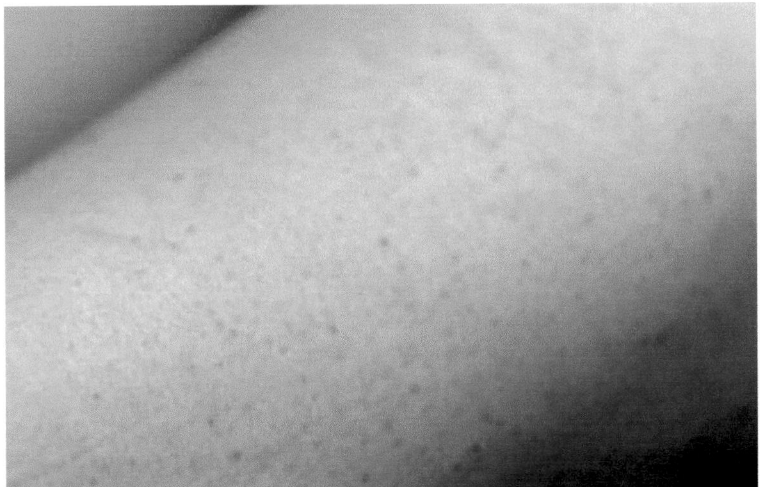

Photograph 16: Scurvy causes easy bleeding and bruising, but it often presents with small haemorrhages around the hair follicles of the thighs and bleeding from the gums before large ecchymoses occur.
Bleeding into the skin can cause pinpoint sized lesions, as shown in these pictures or ecchymoses. Ecchymoses are skin lesions caused by bleeding into the skin that are greater in width than five millimetres, petechiae or less than five millimetres. Petechiae and ecchymoses are flat and do not blanch with pressure. Bleeding into the tissues is very common in anorexia nervosa, but less frequent in bulimia nervosa. If bruising is tender it is likely unrelated to the eating disorder. Haemoglobin is broken down into bilirubin then biliverdin so the ecchymosis changes colour from red to yellow to green over 5–10 days.

Table 3.2 *(cont.)*

Acrocyanosis Lanugo hair Areas of hyperpigmentation Russell's sign Clubbing Self-injury signs (burn or slash marks, raccoon eyes, hair loss, bruises, needle tracks)	Raynaud's means that there are phases of colour change of the extremities. They may turn one, two or three of the colours white, purple and deep red, in that order. Hyperpigmentation over an area of the trunk can be caused by repeated exposure to heat. This is called erythema ab igne. It occurs if the patient attempts to warm themselves by applying heat to their skin (e.g., hot water bottle or radiator). Clubbing in anorexia nervosa is usually due to abuse of laxatives. However, it can be due to other diseases, including sprue and Graves' disease.
Neurological Muscle strength Sensation (touch, joint position sense, temperature sense) Reflexes (delayed relaxation phase of ankle jerk) Chvostek's sign Trousseau's sign Lateral peroneal nerve tap sign	A symmetrical proximal weakness is due to a myopathy. This usually results from a deficiency in potassium, magnesium, phosphate or calcium. Chvostek's sign is the involuntary contraction of the seventh cranial nerve elicited by tapping over it, where it passes through the parotid gland in front of the ear. Trousseau's sign is the involuntary contraction of the hand caused by cutting off blood flow to the hand and arm by elevating the pressure in a blood pressure cuff fastened around the arm, above the systolic pressure and waiting, until the hand goes into spasm or discomfort occurs (maximum time five minutes). The lateral peroneal nerve tap sign is the involuntary dorsiflexion of the foot caused by tapping on the lateral peroneal nerve where it crosses the neck of the fibula

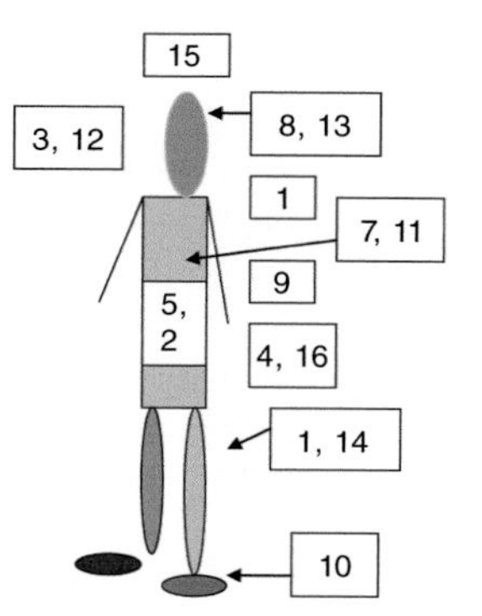

1. *w**A**sting*
2. *la**N**ugo hair*
3. *hyp**O**thermia*
4. ***R**ussell's sign*
5. *hyp**E**rcarotenaemia*
6. ***X**erosis*
7. *m**I**tral valve prolapse*
8. *p**A**rotid hypertrophy*
9. *late**N**t tetany*
10. *d**E**layed relaxation of the tendon jerks*
11. *b**R**adyacardia*
12. ***V**olume depletion*
13. ***O**rganic brain syndrome*
14. *brui**S**ing*
15. *h**A**ir loss*

Figure 3.1 Signs of eating disorders mnemonic.

Measuring Weight, Height, and Estimating Body Fat

Study Questions

- **How can you estimate a patient's goal/ideal/best weight?**
- **How can you best follow the increase in body fat in refeeding?**

Table 3.3 summarises the benefits and limitations of commonly used methods. Of these, body mass index (BMI) is most often used to monitor a patient's response to refeeding. The steps needed to obtain an accurate BMI are measuring height, measuring weight, and calculating the BMI.

Measuring the Height

- Measure height with the patient standing, using a stadiometer or portable anthropometer.
- Shoes or socks should not be worn.
- Clothing that allows the patient's posture to be seen should be worn.
- The back and head should be straight with the patient's eyes looking forward.
- The feet, knees, buttocks, and shoulder blades should be in contact with the vertical surface of the stadiometer, anthropometer, or wall.
- The arms should be hanging loosely at the sides with palms facing the thighs.
- The patient should take a deep breath and stand tall to help straighten their spine.
- Lower the movable headpiece gently, until it just touches the crown of the head.
- Read the height in meters.

Measuring the Weight

- Use the same scale each time (preferably one with sliding weights along the top, as used in hospitals and gymnasiums, because these scales are the most accurate (balance beam scale).
- The balance should be placed on a hard, flat surface.
- Ensure the scale is calibrated accurately at zero before use.
- Measure the weight before a meal.
- The patient should stand unassisted, as still as possible, in the middle of the platform.
- Read the weight and record in kilograms.

Patients with anorexia nervosa may attempt to increase their weight by wearing heaving clothing, strapping weights close to their body, carrying heavy objects in their pockets, stepping unevenly on the scale, binging before being weighed (only to purge later), or drinking excessive amounts of water and avoiding urinating before being weighed. To increase the sensitivity to measure a change in weight, weigh at the same time of the day, preferably in the morning, immediately after voiding, without excess clothing (no coat, scarf, shoes, belt, watch, or jewellery).

Calculating the BMI

The BMI is the most commonly used way to measure the extent to which a patient is underweight or overweight. The BMI can be calculated by dividing the patient's weight in kilograms, by the square of his or her height in meters, as indicated by the formula in Figure 3.2.

Table 3.3 Measuring body weight/fat

Test	Tool	Weight	Body fat	Lean mass	Reliability	Limitations	Cost	Availability
Anthropometrics	Skinfold callipers	No	Yes	No, but can follow mid-arm circumference	Low to high	Very observer dependent	Low	Limited
Body mass index	Scale and stadiometer	Yes	No	No	High	Does not measure body compartments	Low	Very
DEXA	DEXA machine	No	Yes	Yes	High	Expensive and radiation exposure	High	Limited
CT scan of whole body	CT scanner	No	Yes	Yes	High	Cost and radiation exposure	Very High	Limited
BIA	BIA machine	No	Yes	Yes	Low	The result is highly dependent on body water	Moderate	Limited

BIA, bioelectrical independence analysis; CT, computed tomography; DEXA, dual x-ray absorptiometry.

$$BMI = \frac{weight\ (kg)}{[height\ (m)]^2}$$

Figure 3.2. How to calculate body mass index.

To calculate BMI, weight must be in kilograms and height must be in meters. The BMI is used because of its convenience, but it has limitations:

- It is difficult to use in young children who are growing or whose height is stunted by illness.
- It gives no indication of body composition. For example, an athlete with increase muscle may be in a 'normal' range of BMI, despite having a very low total body fat.

BMI Percentiles

To determine whether children, young adolescents, and short people are growing normally, the BMI percentile should be followed over time, rather than the BMI itself. Change in a patient's percentile (e.g., decreasing from the fiftieth percentile to the fifth percentile) is a more accurate indicator of malnutrition than BMI.

Anthropometry

Estimating total body fat by anthropometry can be an accurate, reliable, and inexpensive. However, without training and experience, anthropometric measurements are not reliable. An experienced colleague can provide the training required. The most important methodology to learn is how to locate the measurement sites and how much tissue to 'pinch'. The callipers should measure the thickness of the skin and subcutaneous tissue, not muscle and not only skin.

How to Measure Skinfolds

- Always take all measurements on the left side of the body (or the same side if the patient has no left arm).
- When using the callipers to measure skinfolds, pick up the skin and subcutaneous tissue (subcutaneous fat). Take care not to pick up the underlying muscle or just the skin.
- Measure the midarm circumference, biceps, and triceps skinfolds with the arm held straight forward and parallel to the ground, and with the forearm bent upward at a right angle (90 degrees).
- Measure the subscapular and suprailiac skinfolds with the arms hanging loosely at the sides and the shoulders relaxed.
- Locate the midarm point by halving the distance between the olecranon and the acromion (Figure 3.3).
- **Midarm circumference**: measure the midarm circumference at the midarm point with the muscles relaxed.
- **Biceps skinfold:** measure the biceps skinfold at the midarm point, with the callipers pointing vertically downward (Figure 3.4).
- **Triceps skinfold:** measure the triceps skinfold at the midarm point, from below the arm, with the callipers pointing vertically upward (Figure 3.5).

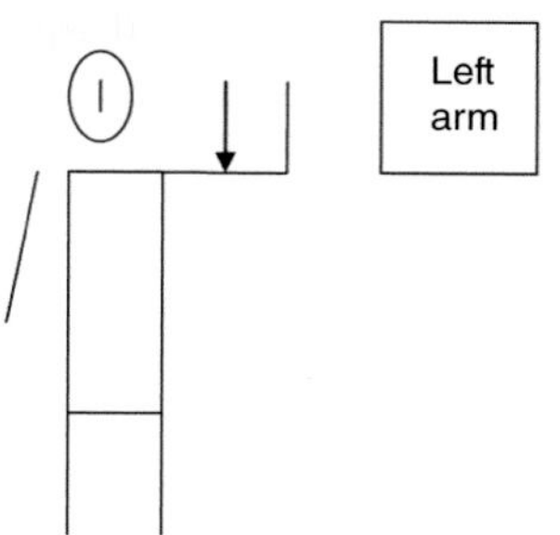

Mid-arm point is half way between the olecranon (knob at elbow) and the acromion (hollow when you lift your shoulder). Position the arm at a right angle to the body and the forearm at a right angle to the arm.

Figure 3.3 The midarm point.

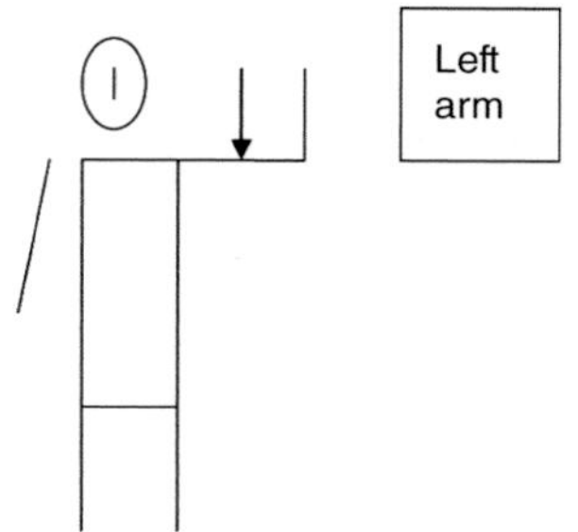

Biceps skinfold is measured at the midarm point with the callipers pointing directly downwards.

Figure 3.4 The biceps skinfold.

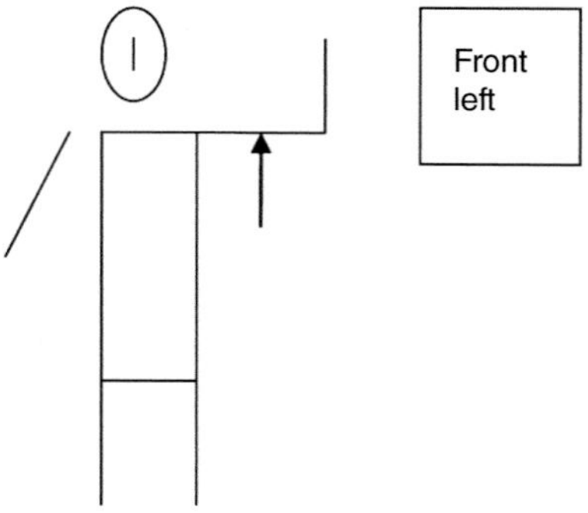

Triceps skinfold is measured at the midarm point with the callipers pointing directly upwards.

Figure 3.5 The triceps skinfold.

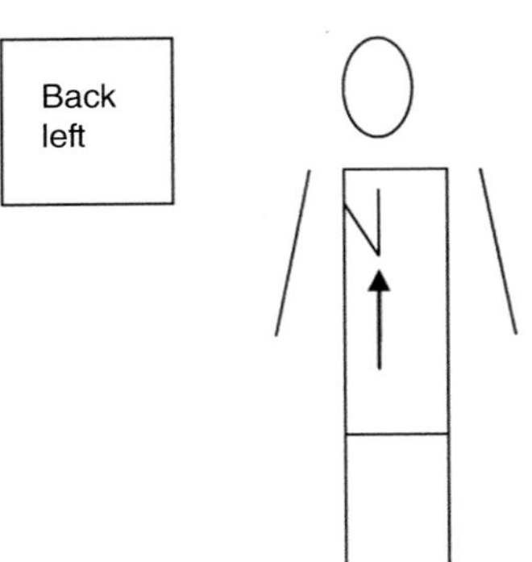

Subscapular skinfold is measured at the lower tip of the scapula (wing-shaped bone on upper back) with the callipers pointing directly upwards.

Figure 3.6 The subscapular skinfold.

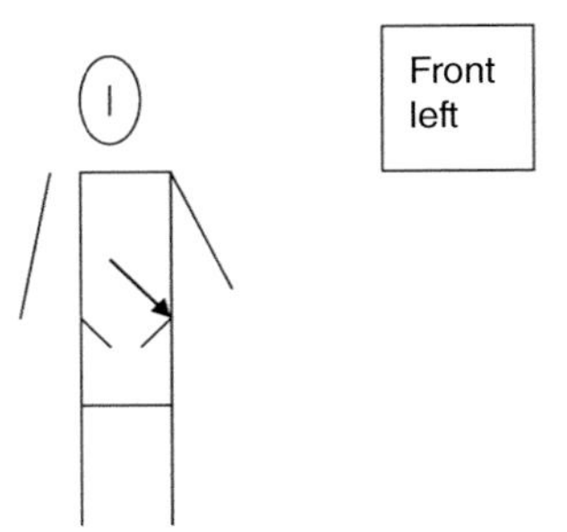

Suprailiac skinfold is measured just anterior to the boney prominence (anterior superior iliac spine) about half way down the abdomen.

Figure 3.7 The suprailiac skinfold.

- **Subscapular skinfold:** measure the subscapular skinfold at the tip of the scapula, with the callipers held horizontally (Figure 3.6).
- **Suprailiac skinfold**: measure the suprailiac skinfold just medial to the anterior superior iliac crest, with the callipers held horizontally (Figure 3.7).

Estimating Total Body Fat with Skinfold Measurements

1. Take the sum of the biceps (B), triceps (T), subscapular (SC) and suprailiac (SI) skinfold measurements: B + T + SC + SI = Total skinfolds.
2. Estimate the total body fat using the total skinfolds and the Durnin and Womersley Table. (http://journals.cambridge.org/action/displayAbstract?fromPage=online&aid=837064; Table 3.4).

Table 3.4 Durnin and Womersely table[a]

Skinfolds (mm)	Males (age in years)				Females (age in years)			
	17–29	30–39	40–49	≥50	16–29	30–39	40–49	≥50
15	4.8	–	–	–	10.5	–	–	–
20	8.1	12.2	12.2	12.6	14.1	17.0	19.8	21.4
25	10.5	14.2	15.0	15.6	16.8	19.4	22.2	24.0
30	12.9	16.2	17.7	18.6	19.5	21.8	24.5	26.6
35	14.7	17.7	19.6	20.8	21.5	23.7	26.4	28.5
40	16.4	19.2	21.4	22.9	23.4	25.5	28.2	30.3
45	17.7	20.4	23.0	24.7	25.0	26.9	29.6	31.9
50	19.0	21.5	24.6	26.5	26.5	28.2	31.0	33.4
55	20.1	22.5	25.9	27.9	27.8	29.4	32.1	34.6
60	21.2	23.5	27.1	29.2	29.1	30.6	33.2	35.7
65	22.2	24.3	28.2	30.4	30.2	31.6	34.1	36.7
70	23.1	25.1	29.3	31.6	31.2	32.5	35.0	37.7
75	24.0	25.9	30.3	32.7	32.2	33.4	35.9	38.7
80	24.8	26.6	31.2	33.8	33.1	34.3	36.7	39.6
85	25.5	27.2	32.1	34.8	34.0	35.1	37.5	40.4
90	26.2	27.8	33.0	35.8	34.8	35.8	38.3	41.2
95	26.9	28.4	33.7	36.6	35.6	36.5	39.0	41.9
100	27.6	29.0	34.4	37.4	36.4	37.2	39.7	42.6
105	28.2	29.6	35.1	38.2	37.1	37.9	40.4	43.3
110	28.8	30.1	35.8	39.0	37.8	38.6	41.0	43.9
115	29.4	30.6	36.4	39.7	38.4	39.1	41.5	44.5
120	30.0	31.1	370	40.4	39.0	39.6	42.0	45.1
125	30.5	31.5	37.6	41.1	39.6	40.1	42.5	45.7
130	31.0	31.9	38.2	41.8	40.2	40.6	43.0	46.2
135	31.5	32.3	38.7	42.4	40.8	41.1	43.5	46.7
140	32.0	32.7	39.2	43.0	41.3	41.6	44.0	47.2
145	32.5	33.1	39.7	43.6	41.8	42.1	44.5	47.7
150	32.9	33.5	40.2	44.1	42.3	42.6	45.0	48.2
155	33.3	33.9	40.7	44.6	42.8	43.1	45.4	48.7
160	33.7	34.3	41.2	45.1	43.3	43.6	45.8	49.2
165	34.1	34.6	41.6	45.6	43.7	44.0	46.2	49.6
170	34.5	34.8	42.0	46.1	44.1	44.4	46.6	50.0

Table 3.4 *(cont.)*

Skinfolds (mm)	Males (age in years)				Females (age in years)			
	17–29	30–39	40–49	≥50	16–29	30–39	40–49	≥50
175	34.9	–	–	–	–	44.8	47.0	50.4
180	35.3	–	–	–	–	45.2	47.4	50.8
185	35.6	–	–	–	–	45.6	47.8	51.2
190	35.9	–	–	–	–	45.9	48.2	51.6
195	–	–	–	–	–	46.2	48.5	52.0
200	–	–	–	–	–	46.5	48.8	52.4
205	–	–	–	–	–	–	49.1	52.7
210	–	–	–	–	–	–	49.4	53.0

[a] The equivalent fat content, as a percentage of body weight, for a range of values for the sum of four skinfolds (biceps, triceps, subscapular, and suprailiac) of males and females of different ages. In two-thirds of the instances, the error was within ±3.5 per cent of the body weight as fat for the women and ±5.0 per cent for the men.

How to Use the Durnin and Womersley Table

1. Select the male or female section. For patients who are undergoing sex change, continue to use the sex from which they are changing for six months and then switch to their new gender. Testosterone and oestrogen cause a gradual change in body fat and lean body mass.
2. Select the correct age range column, according to the patient's age.
3. The per cent total body fat is found where the row (total skinfolds) crosses the correct column (Table 3.4).
4. If the total skinfolds lies between two rows of the chart, the total body fat falls within the range where those rows cross the correct column. Estimate the total body fat using interpolation (see Interpolation).
5. If the total skinfold falls below the chart, estimate the total body fat using extrapolation (see Extrapolation).

Interpolation

Example: A girl aged 18 years has a total skinfold of 17.5 mm. This falls between the 15-mm and 20-mm rows on the Durnin and Womersley Table. Steps:

1. Calculate what fraction of the interval the total skinfolds takes up. Calculate the fraction by dividing the difference between the total skinfolds and the first row below them (17.5 mm – 15 mm = 2.5 mm) by the interval (5 mm): 2.5 mm/5 mm = 0.5 mm.
2. Determine the per cent body fat in the total interval in question. In this example, between the rows for 20 mm and 15 mm the body fat range is: 14.1% body fat – 10.5% body fat = 3.6% body fat.

3. To estimate the per cent body fat, you must add to the bottom row, multiply the fraction from step 1, and the per cent total body fat from step 2: 0.5 × 3.6% body fat = 1.8% total body fat.
4. Finally, the total per cent body fat is calculated by adding the per cent body fat in the range calculated in step three to the per cent body fat on the table at the lowest part of the range: 10.5% body fat + 1.8% body fat = 12.3% total body fat.

Extrapolation

Extrapolation is the same as interpolation, except extrapolation is used for values that fall below the table. Extrapolation does not provide an accurate estimate of the per cent body fat, although the reliability and sensitivity to change is high. Estimates of total body fat obtained by extrapolation should be used to determine whether body fat is increasing, decreasing, or remaining the same, but not as an accurate estimate of actual body fat.

What Equipment Is Needed to Measure Skinfolds?

Use a soft measuring tape (like a sewing tape) to measure length and circumference. Use callipers to measure skinfold thickness. Harpenden callipers are more accurate than Lange callipers. Good quality Harpenden callipers are expensive, but they are accurate, reliable, and durable. They should be kept in their box between uses to protect the spring and gauge.

Bioelectrical Impedance Analysis

Various commercial devices estimate total body fat using measurements of the electrical conductivity and resistance of the body. Bioelectrical impedance analysis uses algorithms that vary between devices and also requires weight and other information to estimate body fat. Electricity is not conducted by fat, because adipose tissue (fat) is less than five per cent water, whereas lean tissue is a good conductor of electricity, because it is mostly water. Bioelectrical impedance estimates the proportion of the body that is adipose tissue by measuring how much electricity is conducted by the body. Unfortunately, this method of estimating total body fat is unreliable in patients with any excess or deficiency of fluid, as is common in patients with eating disorders. As well, the algorithms used to estimate body fat are not accurate in low weight subjects.

Dual-Energy X-Ray Absorptiometry

Dual-energy x-ray absorptiometry (DEXA) is the standard method used to estimate total body fat in nutritional research. DEXA can also estimate the amount of body fat in a body region, but not with the precision of computed tomography (CT) or magnetic resonance imaging. The clinical usefulness of DEXA is limited by radiation exposure and limited availability.

CT Scanning

CT scanning accurately measures the amount and distribution of body fat. It is often used to measure abdominal fat in a cross-section of the body, increased abdominal fat is a risk factor for atherosclerosis. A CT scan is not used for total body fat estimation because it is costly and exposes the patient to a large dose of radiation.

Magnetic Resonance Imaging

Magnetic resonance imaging accurately measures the amount and distribution of body fat. Unlike CT, it uses magnetism (not radiation); it is more costly and is therefore rarely used to measure total body fat.

Implications for Health Care Professionals

Most clinicians do not use anthropometry. They use weight and height measurements and calculate BMI. BMI was developed to stratify weight by height for population research – not for individual measurement. It may be preferable to record and discuss weight alone because it may be more difficult for the patient and your staff to understand the variability in measurements owing to urination, defecation, eating, drinking, sweating, and the weight of clothing when discussing the BMI, which has a somewhat magical quality for many. One must constantly remind oneself of the normal variability in weight to avoid reinforcing the fear of weight gain.

Patient Explanation

- In measuring your weight, your health professional will use the method with which they are most familiar. This is good.
- Remember that all measurements are estimates of a true value. Look for trends over two or three weeks. Discuss your concerns with your health care professional.

Chapter 4

Complications by System

Study and Questions

- *A patient says they are experiencing palpitations during a session. What will you do?*
- *A patient's mother phones saying her son collapsed behind the steering wheel of her car when driving? What is your approach?*
- *How does a patient become aware he or she has osteoporosis/osteopenia?*
- *Can patients with an eating disorder (ED) be immunised (vaccinated)? Does it work?*

Nervous System

Case: If a patient collapses and loses consciousness what is your plan?

The Brain (Central Nervous System)

Death of Cells at the Base of the Brain (Central Pontine Myelolysis)

Brain cells can die if a serum sodium that is very low is elevated too quickly in a malnourished patient. Therefore, if you have a patient who has a very low serum sodium – correct it slowly – over days not hours.

A stroke (cerebrovascular accident) can occur in anorexia nervosa (AN) if a blood clot from a leaky heart valve (mitral valve prolapse) dislodges and blocks a blood vessel in the brain. This complication is rare. It can also occur if a clot dislodging from an infection of the heart value (bacterial endocarditis) after dental work done performed without antibiotics. In patients with AN who have a leaky heart valve (mitral valve prolapse), antibiotics should be given before for all medical procedures that can cause bacteria to be released into the blood (i.e., those involving the mouth, bowel, bladder, or infections).

Drowsiness or Loss of Consciousness (Decreased Level of Consciousness)

Drowsiness or loss of consciousness (decreased level of consciousness) is most commonly due to low blood sugar (hypoglycaemia) and should be treated immediately as if it is hypoglycaemia, whether you know it is or not. However, it can also be due to overdose of drugs whether intentional or not, low body temperature (hypothermia), decreased blood flow to the brain caused by a heart arrhythmia, death of brain cells in the base of the brain (central pontine myelolysis), low serum sodium (hyponatremia), seizures, or head injury.

Table 4.1 Causes of seizures

Classification	Cause	Investigations	Special treatment
Metabolic	Hypoglycaemia Alkalaemia Hypomagnesaemia Hypocalcaemia Hyponatraemia	Blood glucose Screening bicarbonate Serum magnesium low, calcium low, sodium (low or rapid change in level)	Correct abnormality Do not treat a single seizure with antiseizure medications
Cerebral hypoperfusion	Dysrhythmia Vasovagal attack Postural hypotension	Postural blood pressure changes History of typical symptoms of a vasovagal attack Holter monitor	Prevent cerebral hypoperfusion Cardiological consultation
Lowered seizure threshold	Medications (e.g., bupropion), medication withdrawal (e.g., benzodiazepines, barbiturates), alcohol withdrawal	Medication record	Benzodiazepines should be restarted and tapered at no more than 20% a day Alcohol withdrawal usually only has one seizure so do not treat with medications for epilepsy

Seizures

Seizures in patients with an ED are usually caused by low blood sugar (hypoglycaemia) or withdrawal from prescribed or recreational medications (Table 4.1). They can also be caused by low serum magnesium (hypomagnesemia) or low serum sodium (hyponatremia).

Seizure-Like Episodes of Psychological Origin (Pseudoseizures)

Seizure-like episodes of psychological origin (pseudoseizures) are rare in patients with EDs. You can distinguish pseudoseizures from seizures by measuring a serum prolactin, which is normal after a pseudoseizure but elevated after a seizure. One-third of patients with pseudoseizures also have seizures.

Confusion (Organic Brain Syndrome)

Confusion (organic brain syndrome) can be caused by severe malnutrition (protein calorie malnutrition), medications or recreational drugs, deficiencies of magnesium, calcium, phosphorus, thiamine, vitamin B_{12}, low serum sodium (hyponatraemia), too much vitamin A (vitamin A toxicity), swelling or shrinking (crenation) of the brain owing to fluid shifts, seizures, and loss of the ability to form new memories owing to thiamine deficiency (Wernicke's encephalopathy). Shrinking of the brain (pseudoatrophy) is usually due to fluid shifts. Neuropsychological testing can return to normal in as little as six to twelve weeks if confusion is only due to malnutrition. The diagnosis of a reduction in brain size diagnosed by a radiologist usually has no significance and returns to normal with treatment. Do not tell the patient that their brain has shrunk, because this may produce marked anxiety and depression.

Spinal cord

Vitamin B_{12} deficiency can cause dysfunction of the spinal cord (subacute combined degeneration), resulting in a decreased ability to determine the movement and position of joints in the body (decreased joint position sense), decreased ability to feel vibration (decreased vibration sense), and weakness (upper motor neuron weakness).

Muscle

Weakness of the muscle itself (myopathy) can be due to a deficiency of magnesium, calcium, potassium, phosphorus, vitamin C, or general malnutrition. The muscle weakness is usually in the big muscles of the arms and legs (proximal muscles) and reverses with supplementation if it is due to a deficiency.

Many drugs can cause muscle weakness including major tranquilisers (olanzapine, quetiapine), drugs that increase serotonin in the brain (serotoninergic syndrome), ipecac, and ondansetron. Drug toxicity can also be caused by an interaction between medications, neither of which would have caused the weakness themselves.

Weakness of the organ muscles (smooth muscle wasting, e.g., of the diaphragm, heart, bowel, bladder) is usually caused by malnutrition (protein–calorie malnutrition), but magnesium deficiency can cause reversible smooth muscle weakness. Magnesium deficiency results in weakness of the muscles of the eyes responsible for focusing on objects that are near (ciliary muscles of the eye), so magnesium deficiency decreases the patient's ability to maintain visual focus (e.g., computer screen or book) at the same time as it causes weakness of the limbs. Smooth muscles take many months or years to normalise after weight restoration, in contrast with the skeletal muscles that can recover in weeks to months.

Severe phosphate deficiency causes immediate weakness of all muscles in the body, including the heart, and results in acute congestive heart failure.

Peripheral Nerves

Peripheral neuropathy can occur when a nerve is compressed or due to deficiency of vitamin B_{12}, pyridoxine, malnutrition itself (protein–calorie malnutrition), as well as an excess of B vitamins. A specialised test called a nerve conduction study can diagnose a peripheral neuropathy by demonstrating that the nerve does not conduct electricity normally.

A pressure neuropathy occurs when superficial nerves are compressed owing to less padding from loss of fatty or other tissue around it, or owing to loss of consciousness that results in continued compression of the nerve. Foot drop is caused by continued pressure on the outside of the lower leg (the peroneal nerve) and a tingling or bothersome feeling on the thigh (neuralgia paresthetica) is caused by pressure on the groin (the lateral femoral cutaneous nerve) owing to prolonged pressure sometimes seen when yoga positions are held too long.

Frequency of Complications

Common: confusion (organic brain syndrome) is common with very low weight as are muscles weakness, organ muscle weakness, and decreased size of the muscles.

Uncommon: reduced size of the brain on brain imaging (pseudoatrophy of the brain), nerve dysfunction (pressure neuropathy), seizures, lowered level of consciousness, loss of short-term memory (Wernicke's encephalopathy).

Rare: (cerebrovascular accidents), death of brain cells at the base of the brain (central pontine myelolysis), spinal column dysfunction owing to vitamin B_{12} deficiency (subacute combined degeneration).

Implications for Health Care Professionals

- Treat confusion or decreased level of consciousness as hypoglycaemia until proved otherwise.
- Do not correct low serum sodium levels quickly. This action will prevent death of brain cells at the base of the brain (central pontine myelolysis). Serum sodium should be corrected over many days.
- Give antibiotic prophylaxis to low weight patients with AN and heart murmur (mitral valve prolapse), especially before dental procedures.
- Muscle weakness with associated cramping is usually due to magnesium deficiency, even when the serum magnesium is normal. If the patient cannot maintain the focus of their eyes when reading or using a computer, they likely have a magnesium deficiency.
- Patients will complain of shortness of breath with exertion up to a year or two after recovery owing to smooth muscle atrophy of their diaphragms. Maximal inspiratory pressure and the maximal expiratory pressure tests performed in a pulmonary function laboratory will confirm the diagnosis.
- The patient may be unable to understand even simple concepts owing to an organic brain syndrome caused by the malnutrition. Supportive psychotherapy is best until the patient's cognition has improved.
- Pseudoatrophy of the brain (brain shrinkage seen on the computed tomography (CT) scan or MRI) is likely due to dehydration. This will reverse when the dehydration is corrected.
- When the patient is most malnourished, and particularly when they are sedated, attention must be given to preventing pressure sores of their skin and pressure damage to their nerves. Pressure neuropathies are most common over the ulnar nerve at the elbow, the radial nerve behind the upper arm, and the lateral peroneal nerve where it crosses the neck of the fibula.

Patient Explanation

- Muscle weakness is usually due to malnutrition. Gaining weight will reverse it. Occasionally, it is due to vitamin or mineral deficiencies. Blood tests are needed to diagnose these deficiencies. A deficiency is treated by giving you the vitamin and mineral that you are deficient in.
- If your body weight is low, your brain will not function properly. Your memory and concentration will be impaired. Depression, anxiety, and obsessive-compulsive thinking will be worsen and the benefit of medications will be less at low body weight.

Dental

EDs can cause erosion and staining of the teeth, gum recession, and friability and bleeding, and result in tooth loss. Decalcification of the lingual, palatal, and posterior occlusive surfaces of the teeth is referred to as perimylolysis and results from erosion by gastric acid during vomiting. Amalgams are resistant to acid, so they become more obvious as enamel erosion progresses. The patient may complain of increased temperature sensitivity of their teeth and develop caries more frequently.

Patients with AN get viral infections less frequently than normal people and bacterial and fungal infections at the same frequency as people in good health. However, their response to bacterial and fungal infections is impaired. In addition, their symptoms from the infection are delayed and decreased, including fever, pain, and elevated white count – by days to a couple of weeks. Dental or other infection must, therefore, be suspected with far fewer clues than in other patients. Patients may present with huge abscesses of their mandible or large fungal infections in the dental area with few symptoms.

Mitral valve prolapse with regurgitation can develop in patients with AN and increases as the heart size and shape reduce and change. If this occurs, antibiotic prophylaxis should be given before dental procedures.

Scurvy (vitamin C deficiency) is uncommon, but not rare in AN. It causes swollen and bleeding gums and is usually associated with perifollicular haemorrhages on the thighs.

Frequency of Complications

Usual: mild erosion of the teeth, increased frequency of caries.

Common: erosion of the teeth with tender teeth and gum recession.

Uncommon: severe erosion of the teeth, gum recession, staining of the teeth, and loss of teeth.

Implications for Health Care Professionals

Tooth and gum disease are common in patients with AN, particularly when associated with vomiting. Patients should be taught the details about dental complications. For many young people, staining and loss of teeth are huge motivation to recovery. Tell the patient that, if they vomit, they should rinse their mouth immediately afterward, but delay tooth brushing for half an hour because brushing will remove some of the tooth matrix that is unstable during that time. The patient should consult a dentist every six months for treatment and prevention. If the patient says they are uncomfortable telling the dentist they vomit, they can tell the dentist they have severe heart burn (oesophageal reflux).

Patient Information

- Tooth and gum disease is caused by malnutrition, poor eating, bingeing, and especially by vomiting. After vomiting, wait 30 minutes before brushing your teeth.
- Tooth and gum disease can be lessened by improving nutrition, reducing or stopping vomiting, and ensuring good dental hygiene, including rinsing the mouth after vomiting and regular dental check-ups. If you are too embarrassed to tell your dentist you have an ED, then tell them you have heartburn.

- If your doctor tells you that your heart has a leaky valve, ask whether you need to have antibiotics before dental and medical procedures. If so, you should warn your dentist beforehand or the procedure may have to be cancelled at the last minute.

Skin

Case

A 28-year-old woman with AN presented with multiple lesions on her face. She reported having lanced her face with needles to drain the lesion. However, the rash grew and became painful. Investigations revealed fungi within the sores on her face.

The cutaneous manifestations of AN depend upon three factors: the nutritional and caloric content of the foods ingested and omitted, purging techniques, and illness duration (Table 4.2). Both protein–calorie malnutrition and specific nutritional deficiencies are responsible for many of the cutaneous signs of AN. Unless otherwise indicated, feeding and correction of deficiencies are the specific treatments required.

Dry Skin

Dry skin, or xerosis, is seen in most undernourished patients. Xerosis is usually secondary to a deficiency of vitamins and trace elements and may be associated with the sick euthyroid syndrome commonly seen in AN. Xerosis is exacerbated by frequent washing, which may indicate concomitant obsessive-compulsive disorder. Xerosis can be reduced with moisturising ointments and creams, but will not resolve fully without adequate nutrition.

Lanugo Hair

Lanugo hair (hypertrichosis) is fine hair that is caused by the severe protein–calorie malnutrition of AN. It is not caused by starvation from other causes. Lanugo hair is distributed primarily on the back, abdomen, and forearms and presents as fine, downy, soft hairs that are darker in dark-skinned patients. It resolves with restoration of normal total body fat. The diagnosis of lanugo hair is established clinically. Histologically, lanugo hair is indistinguishable from normal hair.

Hair Loss (Telogen Effluvium)

Hair loss in AN is usually due to rapid shedding of old hairs – that regrow. Telogen effluvium (TE) is the generalised shedding of normal telogen club hairs and is induced by physical or psychological stress. Growing hairs are called anagen hairs and resting hairs that are ready to be shed are telogen hairs. In TE, some hair follicles are abruptly converted from anagen to telogen. Hair loss develops two to four months after the period of stress, often during episodes of acute weight loss. TE does not continue when the patient's weight stabilises. Examination of the scalp is normal without any inflammation. The hair loss is generalised. Localised hair loss is not due to TE and is most often due to trichotillomania.

Itch (Pruritis)

Causes of pruritus in AN include xerosis, malnutrition-induced dysfunction of cutaneous immunity, or increased opioid activity. The patient may present with cutaneous

Table 4.2 Skin rash in patients with eating disorders

Location	Skin manifestation	Aetiology	Comments
Hair	Trichotillomania	Patchy hair loss owing to patient pulling out own hair. Noninflammatory and nonscarring.	Occasionally present. Treatment with clomipramine is effective in the short term. Hair should grow back once behaviour stops.
	Telogen effluvium	Generalised shedding of normal telogen club hairs induced by physical or psychological stress.	Commonly present. Hair should grow back once stress is resolved.
	Pili torti	Hair shaft abnormality in which individual hairs are twisted up to 360 degrees on their own axis.	Uncommon. May be due to hypercarotenaemia or hypothyroidism.
Nails	Nail dystrophy	Abnormal nail formation in the setting of protein calorie malnutrition and specific deficiencies, including ferritin, B_{12}, folate, zinc, magnesium, calcium, and phosphorus.	Occasionally present. Normal nails likely to grow back slowly once nutritional deficiencies resolved.
	Koilonychia	Spooning of the nails (concave centrally and reflected upwards laterally) owing to iron deficiency. May also be associated with pallor and/or glossitis.	Occasionally present. Serum ferritin measurement recommended. Dietary cause must not be presumed and gastrointestinal symptoms, self-phlebotomy. and faecal occult blood measurement should be considered.
Perioral/ oral	Angular stomatitis	Fissuring of the oral commissure usually associated with riboflavin and other vitamin deficiencies, although fungal infection and habitual tongue licking should be excluded.	Occasionally present. Treatment with multiple vitamin tablets is recommended.
	Acrodermatitis enteropathica (also hands)	Pustules, scaling, and erosions seen on the face and hands owing to zinc deficiency.	Uncommon. Supplementation with oral zinc is an effective treatment.

Table 4.2 *(cont.)*

Location	Skin manifestation	Aetiology	Comments
			Consider that zinc deficiency may occur in the setting of prolonged copper supplementation because copper competes with zinc for absorption.
	Scurvy (also legs)	Gingival hypertrophy and easy bleeding owing to vitamin C deficiency. Also seen in ecchymoses, perifollicular haemorrhages, follicular keratotic plugs, and impaired wound healing.	Uncommon. Associated with anaemia, subperiosteal haemorrhages, deep haemorrhages. and the dehiscence of old wounds. Treat with vitamin C supplementation.
Periorbital	Purpura	Small, red spots (petechiae) around the eyes, in a mask-like distribution. Owing to trauma and breakage of the small blood vessels during forceful vomiting	Commonly present. May be due to other exertions that elevate intrathoracic pressure, such as forceful coughing.
	Subconjunctival haemorrhage	Red eye owing to bleeding beneath the conjunctiva as a result of blood vessel damage owing to forceful vomiting.	Commonly present. Other causes of red eye must be excluded.
Hands	Russell's sign	Small scars or callosities on the back of the hand and digits. Result from repeated rubbing of the skin against the upper incisors when the hand is placed in the mouth to induce vomiting.	Commonly present. Although the scars are not reversible, they may decrease in size when the behaviour is discontinued.
	Pompholyx (neurodermatitis)	Tiny, itchy, fluid-filled vesicles commonly on the lateral aspect of the digits. Precipitated by severe stress associated with AN.	Uncommon.
	Hypercarotenaemia	Yellowing of the skin owing to carotene deposition, often noted on palms and soles. Elevated serum carotene is owing to slowed hepatic breakdown of carotene resulting from	Commonly present. Should be distinguished from other causes of yellow skin, such as jaundice, by the absence of a scleral colour change.

Table 4.2 *(cont.)*

Location	Skin manifestation	Aetiology	Comments
		reduced basal metabolic rate. Aggravated by an increased consumption of carotene found in carrots, squash, and spinach.	Restoration of normal nutritional status will hasten carotene metabolism and bring about resolution.
	Acrocyanosis	Cool hands and feet with purple discolouration associated with delayed capillary refill. Presents in the context of severe protein–calorie malnutrition.	Occasionally present. Should resolve with feeding.
	Acrodermatitis enteropathica (also perioral)	Pustules, scaling, and erosions seen on the face and hands owing to zinc deficiency.	Uncommon. Supplementation with oral zinc is an effective treatment. Consider that zinc deficiency may occur in the setting of prolonged copper supplementation because copper competes with zinc for absorption.
	Perniosis	Flat, red lesions located symmetrically on the ends of the fingers, nose, and ears. Precipitated by exposure to cold.	Uncommon. Generally self-limited. Avoid cold exposure and protect the affected areas.
Trunk/ back	Lanugo hair	Fine, downy hair owing to severe protein–calorie malnutrition of AN. Interestingly, does not appear when starvation is due to other causes.	Common. Resolves with restoration of normal total body fat.
	Drug eruptions	Many various skin eruptions may be associated with medications. Drugs used as a method of purging include laxatives, enemas, emetics, diuretics, herbal remedies, and other diet pills.	Occasionally present High. degree of suspicion of medication abuse is necessary.
	Pellagra (also legs, hands)	Hyperpigmented, scaly plaques in sun-exposed areas (hands, face, shins). Casal's neck lace refers to a	Rare. Dermatitis precedes more severe manifestations, including diarrhoea,

Table 4.2 *(cont.)*

Location	Skin manifestation	Aetiology	Comments
		characteristic plaque located around the neck. Owing to deficiency in niacin (vitamin B_3) or tryptophan.	dementia, and death. Nutritional supplementation.
	Prurigo pigmentosa	Itchy, red papules that evolve into an irregular hyperpigmentation. Affected areas include the back, neck and chest. The cause is unknown.	Rare. Ketosis produced by AN may contribute to the pathogenesis.
	Xerosis (also legs/ calves)	Dry skin owing to deficiency of vitamins and trace elements. May be associated with the sick euthyroid syndrome.	Commonly present. Ameliorated with moisturising ointments and creams, but will not resolve without restoration of normal nutritional status.
Legs/ calves	Scurvy (also oral and any location)	Bruising, perifollicular haemorrhages, and follicular keratotic plugs. Also seen in impaired wound healing, gingival hypertrophy, and easy bleeding. Scurvy is due to vitamin C deficiency.	Uncommon. Associated with anaemia, subperiosteal haemorrhages, deep haemorrhages, and the dehiscence of old wounds. Treat with vitamin C supplementation.
	Oedema	Fluid retention often occurring during refeeding because of low BMR. May also be due to intermittent fluid depletion associated with bingeing and purging, which causes the renin–aldosterone axis to be inappropriately stimulated.	Commonly present. Refeeding oedema is due to fluid shifts and should not be aggressively treated.
	Xerosis (also trunk)	Dry skin owing to deficiency of vitamins and trace elements. May be associated with the sick euthyroid syndrome.	Commonly present. Ameliorated with moisturising ointments and creams, but will not resolve without restoration of normal nutritional status.
	Pellagra (also trunk, hands)	Hyperpigmented, scaly plaques in sun-exposed areas (hands, face, shins). Owing to deficiency in	Rare. Dermatitis precedes more severe manifestations, including diarrhoea,

Table 4.2 *(cont.)*

Location	Skin manifestation	Aetiology	Comments
		niacin (vitamin B_3) or tryptophan.	dementia, and death. Nutritional supplementation.
Any location	Dermatitis artefacta	Bizarrely shaped lesions irregularly scattered over any body surface, owing to self-inflicted harm (slashing, head hitting or burning). Lesions may include excoriations, ulcers, bruising, round-shaped skin excavations, and scars.	Commonly present. Diagnosis of self-harm is difficult because patients are often reluctant to admit to the self-inflicted nature of the lesion. Careful history of depression and suicidal ideation must be obtained and psychological treatment given.
	Self-phlebotomy	Needle track marks present over the veins from which blood has been drawn. The antecubital fossa is the most common location.	Occasionally present. Measurement of serum haemoglobin (because frequent self-phlebotomy can lead to severe anaemia). Treatment with loxapine may reduce this behaviour.
	Erythema ab igne	Irregular hyperpigmented 'lacy' area(s), on any surface area, resulting from the chronic application of hot water bottles or other heating devices by patient s to warm themselves. A constant feeling of cold associated with starvation-induced hypothermia.	Occasionally present. Hyperpigmentation is usually irreversible, despite behaviour modification. Malignant transformation within the patch has been reported.
	Pruritus	Itchy skin and excoriations owing to starvation-induced xerosis, dysfunction of cutaneous immunity, or enhanced levels of opioid activity.	Occasionally present. Rehydration of the skin with ointments and creams and low-dose antihistamines.
	Scurvy (also legs and oral)	Bruising, perifollicular haemorrhages, and follicular keratotic plugs, impaired wound healing, gingival hypertrophy, and easy bleeding. Scurvy is due to vitamin C deficiency.	Uncommonly present. Associated with anaemia, subperiosteal haemorrhages, deep haemorrhages, and the dehiscence of old wounds. Treat with vitamin C supplementation.

lichenification (thickening) and excoriations (scratches) without an identifiable cutaneous abnormality. Therapy includes rehydration of the skin with ointments and creams and low-dose antihistamines.

Hypercarotenaemia (Yellow Skin)

Hypercarotenaemia results from carotene deposition in the tissues causing yellowing of the skin. Elevated serum carotene is due to a lowered basal metabolic rate in AN, with a resultant slowed liver breakdown of carotene. Hypercarotenaemia can be increased by consumption of carotene, found in some foods, including carrots, squash, and spinach. Increased consumption only causes hypercarotenaemia in children and those with liver disease. Only two conditions other than AN cause hypercarotenaemia – hypothyroidism and childhood, both owing to reduced hepatic rate of metabolism of carotene.

The presence of hypercarotenaemia can help to distinguish AN from malabsorption. Serum carotene is low in patients with weight loss owing to malabsorption but high in AN.

Yellow skin owing to hypercarotenaemia can be differentiated from jaundice because hypercarotenaemia causes yellow skin and white eyes, whereas jaundice has yellow skin and yellow eyes. Yellow eyes develop in jaundice because bilirubin binds to the elastin in the eye covering.

Patients can be reassured that hypercarotenaemia has no pathological consequences and that it disappears with weight restoration.

Oedema (Swelling Owing to Excess Fluid)

The low metabolic rate of AN predisposes to fluid retention that causes swelling of tissues owing to excess fluid. Fluid retention can be marked, amounting to more than ten kilograms over a week or two.

Excess fluid is most evident in the dependent parts of the body (those that are lower than the rest of the body). Oedema is therefore most prominent in the feet and ankles of an ambulatory patient or over the sacrum of a bedridden patient. This oedema is pitting oedema. This means that you can make an indentation or pit by pressing with constant moderate pressure, applied by using your finger over a bony prominence in a dependent area, and the pit remains after you stop pressing.

Pitting oedema is not specific to AN. It may also develop in bulimia nervosa (BN), pregnancy, congestive heart failure, and hypoalbuminaemia associated with loss of protein by the kidney, protein loss through the bowel (protein-losing enteropathy), liver disease, and low albumen sometimes seen in patients with AN where there has been severe protein restriction. Usually the serum albumin is normal in AN.

The oedema that occurs during refeeding in AN usually resolves within two weeks if the patient abstains from excess salt and is on bed rest with their legs at the same level of the body without flexing the hips. Hip flexion increases the venous pressure in the legs and can cause oedema and deep venous thrombi.

Refeeding oedema can be limited or prevented by correcting dehydration before or at the very beginning of refeeding. Correcting dehydration decreases the body's marked retention of fluid during refeeding. As an inpatient, if the serum sodium is normal, give intravenous normal saline to normalise the patient's fluid volume. As an outpatient, have the patient drink three cups a day of high-salt Oxo cubes or other drinks that are high in salt. Follow the dehydration treatment protocol. Pressure stockings can be worn if the oedema causes discomfort. Diuretics should be avoided because they result in rebound oedema that can recur over months or years.

Purple Extremities (Acrocyanosis)

Acrocyanosis is cool hands and feet that are violaceous in colour. It is caused by decreased blood flow to and delayed capillary refill from the extremities. It usually occurs in severe protein–calorie malnutrition where the body temperature is low – so the cooler blood of the extremities is prevented from returning to the core of the body by decreasing its flow. It is not associated with any histopathologic abnormalities.

Nail Abnormalities (Nail Dystrophy)

Abnormal nail formation is often seen in protein–calorie malnutrition, as well as with deficiencies of iron, vitamin B_{12}, folate, zinc, magnesium, calcium, and phosphorus. Nail dystrophy may affect the digits unequally, making it difficult to distinguish this from a fungal infection of the nails.

Acne

Acne may develop with weight gain in AN. Tell the patient that weight loss caused them to be hormonally prepubertal, but with weight gain they must go through puberty again, including menses, mood shifts, and acne. Standard treatment is effective for the acne. Interestingly, each time the patient goes through puberty their telomere, that is a genetic marker of their length of life, shortens, thereby shortening their life expectancy.

Spooning of the Nails (Koilonychia)

Koilonychia, also called spooning of the nails, means the nail is deformed with a central concavity, so it looks like a spoon. Koilonychia can occur with iron deficiency and may be associated with pallor and hypochromic microcytic anaemia. However, most patients who are iron deficient do not have koilonychia. Serum ferritin should be measured to confirm the diagnosis of iron deficiency. Iron deficiency can also cause glossitis with flattening of the papillae of the tongue. Iron deficiency is more common if menstruation has persisted and when red meat is not eaten. Rarely, it may be a clue to gastrointestinal pathology like celiac disease. It is necessary to carefully investigate the cause of iron deficiency in all patients. A dietary cause must not be assumed. If there is a history of gastrointestinal symptoms or self-phlebotomy, the cause should be investigated. If iron deficiency presents in a chronic anorexic who is older than forty years, particularly if they are not menstruating, exclude bowel cancer.

Angular Stomatitis

Angular stomatitis, or perleche, is fissuring of the sides of the mouth (oral commissure). It is usually associated with riboflavin and other vitamin deficiencies, but fungal infection and habitual tongue licking are also causes. Laboratory measures of riboflavin are not widely available and riboflavin deficiency is often part of multiple vitamin and mineral deficiencies; therefore, treatment with multiple vitamin tablets is recommended.

Acrodermatitis Enteropathica

Acrodermatitis enteropathica (AE) is the cutaneous manifestations of zinc deficiency. Very dry skin – especially the palms and soles – is the clue to the diagnosis. AE presents as periorificial and acral pustules, scaling, and erosions. There may also be associated changes in taste (dysgeusia), diffuse alopecia, and angular stomatitis. Dysgeusia means a change in taste that may present as decreased taste, change in the taste of foods, a marked preference for certain tastes, or a metallic taste. The pathology of AE reveals acanthosis, parakeratosis, and ballooning degeneration of midepidermal keratinocytes.

Zinc deficiency in AN is usually due to inadequate ingestion of zinc (e.g., especially seafood and cow's milk products). Fibre reduces absorption of zinc by binding it. Zinc deficiency can also be caused by prolonged copper supplementation, because copper competes with zinc for absorption. Zinc deficiency is suggested by skin dryness or rash particularly on the palms and soles, poor skin healing, and dysgeusia but there may have no signs of symptoms.

Supplementation with oral zinc is an effective treatment for zinc deficiency. Zinc can be given as tablets, fifty milligrams of elemental zinc as zinc citrate daily, for three months or until the diet has adequate zinc. Serum zinc does not measure total body or brain zinc. The Accusens-Test for zinc is not reliable. Therefore, zinc supplementation should be given based on symptoms or signs.

Pellagra

Pellagra presents as hyperpigmented and scaly plaques on the hands, face, shins and other sun exposed areas. Casal's necklace refers to a characteristic, well-demarcated, hyperpigmented plaque located around the neck. Pellagra is caused by a deficiency of either niacin (vitamin B_3) or tryptophan. Niacin is a component of the electron transport chain and is essential to glycolysis and other metabolic processes. The dermatitis generally precedes the more severe manifestations of pellagra, which include diarrhoea, dementia, and death. The histopathology of pellagra is indistinguishable from AE.

Scurvy

Scurvy is caused by vitamin C deficiency. Consider scurvy if there is easy bleeding from the gums or tiny haemorrhages around hair follicles on the thighs.

Vitamin C is necessary for the hydroxylation of proline and lysine in collagen biosynthesis. Patients with vitamin C deficiency bleed easily and may develop ecchymoses, gingival hypertrophy, perifollicular haemorrhages, follicular keratotic plugs, and impaired wound healing. Anaemia, subperiosteal haemorrhages, deep haemorrhages, and the dehiscence of old wounds can also occur.

Scurvy is fatal if not treated. Vitamin C blood levels are not widely available so treat early with 500–1,000 milligrams of vitamin C a day for three weeks and then a multiple vitamin containing at least ten milligrams of vitamin C daily.

Skin Complications Caused by Abnormal Behaviour

Erythema Ab Igne

Erythema ab igne is an irregular, fixed, reticulated hyperpigmented patch that is due to the chronic application of hot water bottles or other sources of heat. Patients with AN warm themselves because of a constant feeling of cold caused by the starvation-induced hypothermia. Erythema ab igne can be distinguished histopathologically from other dermatoses only by exclusion. Hyperpigmentation may be irreversible, but even severe hyperpigmentation can decrease if the application of heat is stopped. Rarely, malignant transformation within the patch has been reported. To decrease the likelihood of hyperpigmentation, rotate exposure to warmth to different parts of the body (e.g., abdomen, back, arms, thighs).

Self-Phlebotomy

If a patient with AN self-phlebotomises as a means of losing weight or causing self-harm, needle track marks may be present over the veins from which blood has been drawn. The antecubital fossa is the most common location. Self-phlebotomy can lead to severe anaemia, so the serum haemoglobin should be measured and monitored in patients with anaemia. An unexplained decrease in haemoglobin indicates a high likelihood of self-phlebotomy. Most patients with AN who practice self-phlebotomy are health care professionals. Loxapine is often effective in the treatment of self-phlebotomy.

Self-Inflicted Harm (Dermatitis Artefacta)

Self-inflicted harm includes cutting, slashing, hitting, or burning and may result in bizarre-shaped excoriations, ulcers, bruising, round-shaped skin excavations, and scars anywhere on the body. The diagnosis of self-harm may be difficult because patients are reluctant to admit to or reveal self-inflicted skin lesions. Ecchymoses resemble those of scurvy or coagulopathy, whereas healed cigarette burns on the legs may resemble diabetic dermatopathy. Many patients practice self-harm to dull their emotional pain with physical pain; therefore, once a diagnosis is established, psychological treatment is necessary, and a careful history of depression and suicidal ideation must be obtained.

Compulsive Hair Pulling (Trichotillomania)

Patients with trichotillomania (compulsive hair pulling) have noninflammatory, non-scarring alopecia. The hair loss of trichotillomania characteristically involves only part of the scalp, whereas TE involves the entire scalp. The margins of hair loss in trichotillomania are not distinct, whereas alopecia areata has distinct margins. The hair loss of hyperthyroidism extends from the forehead back towards the temporal area, which is not the distribution of trichotillomania. The histopathology of trichotillomania is distinct, demonstrating trichomalacia. Treatment with clomipramine or other serotonin uptake inhibitors is an effective short-term treatment, but psychological therapy is usually required.

Rare Skin Manifestations

Prurigo Pigmentosa

Prurigo pigmentosa is a rare inflammatory disease of unknown aetiology characterised by pruritic erythematous papules that evolve into a reticular hyperpigmentation. Affected areas include the back, neck, and chest. A case of prurigo pigmentosa has been reported in association with AN. The authors suggest that the ketosis of AN may contribute to the pathogenesis of prurigo pigmentosa.

Pili Torti

There is one report that pili torti, a hair shaft abnormality that results in hair that is twisted up to 360 degrees on its own axis, is present in eighty-two per cent of patients with AN. The authors hypothesised that pili torti is caused by hypercarotenaemia or hypothyroidism in AN.

Perniosis

Perniosis presents as inflammatory, erythematous to violaceous, macules and patches located bilaterally and symmetrically on the proximal phalanges, acral areas, nose, and ears. It develops secondary to an abnormal vascular reaction and is precipitated by exposure to cold. It has been suggested that perniosis in AN is related to altered temperature control and vasoreactivity. Perniosis in AN is usually self-limited and treatment consists of avoiding cold exposure and protection of affected areas.

Neurodermatitis (Pomphylx)

Pomphylx, also known as neurodermatitis, presents as pinpoint, itchy, fluid-filled lumps (vesicles) that are most prominent on the sides of the fingers or toes (lateral aspect of the digits). Histologically, pomphylx is a spongiotic dermatitis with spongiotic vesicle formation. Neurodermatitis is usually precipitated by severe stress.

Eruptive Neurofibromatosis

There has been one report of a rapid worsening of stable neurofibromatosis after the onset of AN.

Signs Associated with Purging Behaviour

Russell's Sign

Gerald Russell, when he made the first description of BN in 1979, noted the presence of calluses over the back of the hand, which resulted from repeated rubbing of the skin against the upper teeth (incisors). The calluses are caused by repeated trauma induced by teeth as the digits of the hand are forced down the throat. There may be one to three scars distributed over the dorsal aspect of the digits and hand. Russell's sign is seen in AN of the purging sub-type as well as BN. Histopathology demonstrates normal scar tissue.

Although the scars are not reversible, they may decrease in size if the causative behaviour is stopped. Occasionally, a dermatologist will inject steroids into the calluses if have recently increased in size in an attempt to decrease their size a little.

Blood under the Skin (Purpura)

When small vessels break under the skin, a pin-sized, blood-coloured lesion results. Petechiae are small, rounded, red or purple spots that are less than three millimetres in size. Purpura are between three millimetres and one centimetre in size. Ecchymoses are larger than one centimetre in size. Both purpura and ecchymoses are usually irregular in shape.

Petechiae are often seen around the eyes (periocular) and may have a mask-like distribution. Purpura may be a sign of scurvy, elevated intrathoracic pressure owing to extreme exertion, or covert self-injection. If the lesions are tender, they may be due to an unrelated vasculitis.

If a group of petechiae or purpura have a precise border, they are likely due to self-injurious behaviour.

Petechiae and purpura are caused by blood and are therefore red or reddish. As the body breaks the blood down into its constituent parts the colour changes from red (blood) to yellow (bilirubin) and finally green (biliverdin). Therefore, a colour change indicates that that the petechiae or purpura are not new.

Subconjunctival Haemorrhage

Forceful vomiting can damage blood vessels in the eye and lead to subconjunctival haemorrhage.

Oedema (Swelling Owing to Excess Fluid)

Binging and purging cause dehydration (see Oedema [Swelling Owing to Excess Fluid] in the section on Skin). To correct this abnormality, the body retains more fluid through the action of the renin–angiotensin–aldosterone axis. If binging and purging continue, the dehydration/fluid retention cycle leads to cyclic oedema. During the fluid retention phase, the oedema causes a rapid increase in body weight that often increases the drive to binge and purge. The cycle oedema will continue to recur until the binge–purge cycle is broken. Angiotensin receptor inhibitors may decrease the amount of fluid retained, but they can cause renal dysfunction and are only effective while being used.

Drug Eruption

Patients with EDs may take medications that are prescribed, over the counter, herbal, or naturopathic, including those that cause purging or weight loss. Medications that cause purging or weight loss include laxatives, enemas, suppositories, emetics, diuretics, herbal remedies, and other diet pills.

Laxative abuse may lead to finger clubbing, thiazide diuretics may cause photosensitivity, ipecac has been implicated in a dermatomyositis-like syndrome, and phenothiazines may cause a fixed drug eruption. Finger clubbing in AN is most commonly associated with chronic use of Senna laxatives and usually reverses if they are stopped.

Other possible drug-related dermatoses may also be seen depending on the patient, drug characteristics, and drug interactions. When taking the medical history, a high degree of suspicion of medication noncompliance, underreport of over-the-counter and recreational drugs, and drug abuse is necessary.

Implications for Health Care Professionals

- Inspect the skin for abnormalities, especially for signs of self-harm. Skin abnormalities often develop during treatment.
- Successful treatment of any skin rash often increases rapport. Patients are usually happy to receive advice and treatment of any skin rash, perhaps because of their low self-esteem about their appearance.
- Refeeding oedema can be limited or prevented by correcting dehydration before refeeding. Give intravenous normal saline to normalise the patient's fluid volume in inpatients before or at the beginning of refeeding – if their serum sodium is not very low. As an outpatient, have the patient drink three cups a day of high-salt Oxo cubes or other drinks that are high in salt a day until their volume status is normal. Measure the patient's volume by their jugular venous pressure and lying to standing blood pressure and heart rate change.
- Iron deficiency: Never assume iron deficiency is dietary – especially if the patient has amenorrhea or older than forty years. Investigate to exclude bowel cancer.
- Zinc can be given as tablets, fifty milligrams elemental zinc as zinc citrate daily, for two months and until the diet has adequate zinc.
- Erythema ab igne: Exposure to localised heat should be rotated to different parts of the body (e.g., abdomen, back, arms, thighs) to decrease the chance of hyperpigmentation.
- An unexplained decrease in haemoglobin suggests the possibility of self-phlebotomy.

Patient Explanation

- Report any new skin rash to the physician.
- A skin rash may be a clue to a deficiency or another disease or complication.
- Acne may develop with weight gain in AN. Weight loss caused your hormones to return to their state before your menses started. With weight gain, your hormones return to the adult state. So you are going through puberty again, including menses, mood shifts, and acne. Standard treatment is effective for the acne. Each time you go through puberty your telomere, which is a genetic marker of your length of life, shortens.
- Erythema ab igne: To decrease the likelihood of dark spots on your skin exposure to localised heat should be rotated to different parts of the body (e.g., abdomen, back, arms, and thighs).

Respiratory

Case

A patient who has recovered from AN sees you in follow-up one year later. She says she feels well except for shortness of breath when jogging.

Lung Function

Weakness of the respiratory muscles in AN is the most common lung abnormality. This weakness results in shortness of breath with aerobic exercise. Respiratory muscle thickness and wasting can be measured by CT scan, but the abnormality is best documented on pulmonary function testing. Order maximal inspiratory pressure and the maximal expiratory pressure measurements to confirm diaphragmatic weakness. Emphysema-like lung changes seen in AN with severe weight loss (vide infra) do not change the results of the routine pulmonary function test. They normalise with weight restoration.

Pulmonary Disorders

Aspiration pneumonia is caused by reflux of stomach contents from the stomach, up the oesophagus, and into the lung. This condition is more likely if there is a history of purging, oesophageal reflux (heartburn), muscular weakness, a decreased level of consciousness, or a nasogastric tube in place. Aspiration pneumonia may be chemical, bacterial, or both. The chest radiograph may remain normal for up to twenty-four hours after aspiration.

Viral infections are less likely in low weight AN. Bacterial and fungal infections are no more likely than in the normal population. However, the body's response to bacterial infections and fungal infection is reduced in AN. As well, symptoms like fever, pain, and increased white blood cell count are delayed. This delays the diagnosis.

If the patient's dentition is poor, suspect an anaerobic pneumonia. Progression to lung abscess and empyema is much more common in AN.

Emphysema-like changes can occur in the lung of patients with AN. This means that there is reduced lung tissue. These changes are not static. They increase as malnutrition worsens and decrease as malnutrition lessens. Any patient with AN who has emphysema-like changes on CT scanning of the lung should not smoke cigarettes. Being diagnosed with emphysema owing to AN is usually a strong motivation for weight gain.

Other Conditions

Spontaneous pneumothorax, pneumomediastinum, and subcutaneous emphysema can occur owing to the extreme elevation of pressure in the chest caused by forceful vomiting.

Frequency of Complications

Common: shortness of breath on exertion owing to wasting of the muscles of respiration, bacterial lung infection.

Uncommon: aspiration pneumonia, bacterial pneumonia that progresses to lung abscess or empyema, pulmonary muscle weakness, spontaneous pneumothorax, subcutaneous emphysema, emphysema-like change in the lung.

Rare: clubbing (if present it is usually caused by concomitant laxative abuse, bacterial endocarditis, or celiac disease).

Implications for Health Care Professionals

Respiratory symptoms in EDs are usually unrelated to the ED. Investigate as usual. However, in low weight AN, bacterial and fungal infections are likely and will present with few symptoms or signs.

Aspiration pneumonia is more likely to occur if the patient has tube feeding or decreased level of consciousness. Aspiration pneumonia may present with cough, shortness of breath, or fever. In AN, the body temperature tends to be subnormal (hypothermia) and fever is less likely or slow to develop. Bacterial infection may be advanced before a fever occurs. An increased level of suspicion for infection and investigation with fewer signs and symptoms than usual is warranted. Abnormalities on chest x-ray may be delayed for twenty-four hours or more in aspiration pneumonia, particularly if there is dehydration.

Cyanosis of the hands and feet is frequent with severe malnutrition, especially with volume depletion. This is caused by desaturation of blood owing to the slow flow (stagnant hypoxia) and is not due to hypoxemia. Central cyanosis (most obvious in the lips) is due to oxygen desaturation of haemoglobin. Central cyanosis is not a characteristic of AN.

Patient Information

- AN does not usually cause disease of the lungs and has no long-term effect on the lungs after weight restoration, except for shortness of breath on exertion owing to wasting of the muscles of the diaphragm that may last for up to two years.
- A blue or purple discolouration at of fingers and or toes may be seen in AN. Treatment is to gain weight and correct dehydration.
- If your doctor says your weight is low, you are more likely to get a bacterial or fungal infection in your body, including your lung. If you do, you will develop a fever and other signs later than if you were a normal weight.

Heart and Blood Vessels

Case

A patient with an ED has been diagnosed with mitral valve prolapse. Her dentist asks whether she needs to take antibiotics before dental procedures.

About one-half of deaths that occur in AN are medical in cause – the most common of them is cardiac arrhythmia. An arrhythmia is more likely if there is hypoglycaemia; QT prolongation; medication use; withdrawal from drugs or alcohol; deficiencies of potassium, magnesium, or phosphate; hypothermia; heart failure; loss of consciousness; or rapid change in heart rate variability (rapid change in the autonomic control of the heart).

Hypoglycaemia is a common and treatable cause of arrhythmia. Hypoglycaemia may present as arrhythmia and loss of consciousness. Hypoglycaemia occurs when liver glycogen stores are low and caloric intake is increased quickly (refeeding). Some people are very aware when they are hypoglycaemic; others are entirely unaware. The hypoglycaemia occurs between thirty minutes and two hours after eating.

Heart rate variability is often prolonged in AN. It is not this prolongation that predisposes to arrhythmia, but rather the rapid decrease in heart rate variability, similar other cardiac diseases like after myocardial infarctions. Heart rate variability can be treated with centrally acting beta-blockers or weight restoration. However, if a patient has markedly increased heart rate variability, they should receive nutrition more slowly. Cardiologists and internists are often unaware of the cardiac complications of EDs and underestimate their importance. To make things worse, critical information about the cause and treatment of arrhythmias in patients with EDs still awaits research.

Cardiac Anatomy

Protein–calorie malnutrition results in wasting of the heart with decreased left ventricular muscle mass, mitral valve prolapse or worsening of pre-existing mitral valve prolapse, and later myofibrillar degeneration of the endocardium. These changes progress slowly over months or years. They reverse with weight gain. They only occur if there is protein–calorie malnutrition and, therefore, do not occur in BN.

A small pericardial effusion may occur, usually if the serum albumin is low. Hypoalbuminemia is infrequent in AN and usually occurs only if the diet is low in both the quality and quantity of protein. The pericardial effusion is diagnosed as an incidental finding on ultrasound examination and rarely causes symptoms or requires treatment.

Cardiac Function

Vitamin and mineral deficiencies can alter cardiac function in AN, BN, or ED not otherwise specified. A deficiency in vitamin B_1 usually causes Wernicke's encephalopathy in patients with EDs. Thiamine requires magnesium and phosphate to be active in humans, so magnesium or phosphorus deficiency can cause thiamine deficiency even after large amounts of thiamine as given the patient. A deficiency in vitamin B_1 (thiamine) can cause wet beriberi with heart failure, but this condition is rare.

Magnesium deficiency can cause arrhythmia, prolongation of the QT interval, or congestive heart failure.

Phosphate deficiency can cause rapid onset of congestive heart failure. During refeeding, serum phosphate levels can decrease rapidly because the body uses a great deal of phosphate during refeeding and the stores of phosphate in the body may be very low. However, complications of phosphate deficiency are unlikely to occur until the serum phosphate level is less than one-half of the lower limit of normal. When phosphate levels decrease, they often decrease slowly at first and then decrease suddenly. Always give supplementary phosphate during refeeding to keep levels in the middle of the normal range.

Deficiency of total body potassium can cause cardiac arrhythmia and worsen congestive heart failure.

A deficiency of selenium can result in heart failure. However, this occurs rarely as the body has large stores of selenium (usually enough to last seventeen years). Deficiencies occur almost exclusively in those who eat produce grown in soil deficient in selenium, such as in New Zealand, China, and British Columbia.

Anaemia caused by folic acid, vitamin B_{12}, iron, or copper deficiency will increase the work of the heart and worsen congestive heart failure. Heart-related physical signs of EDs are shown in Figure 4.1.

Heart Failure

Heart failure is usually due to weakness of the cardiac muscle. Heart failure presents with shortness of breath on exertion accompanied by decreased exercise capacity and increased fatigue. As heart failure worsens, it takes less exertion to cause shortness of

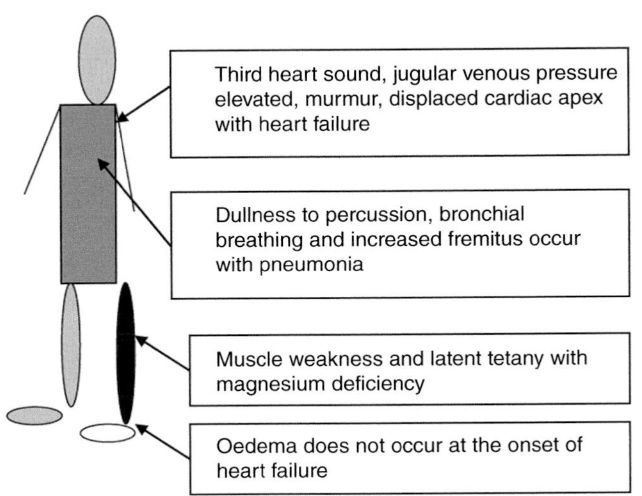

Figure 4.1 Heart/lung sequalae of an eating disorder.

breath, until it is present at rest. Clinical signs of heart failure include increased venous pressure, oedema, and a third heart sound. Important laboratory tests that are helpful to confirm the diagnosis and rule out other causes are the electrocardiogram, the chest radiograph, and echocardiography.

Heart failure in AN is usually of sudden onset and owing to phosphate deficiency. The young patient with heart failure and AN will suddenly be short of breath, have to sit upright to breath, have a rapid heart rate, and have chest wheezing (so called cardiac asthma) rather than the usual basal crackles. This is a life-threatening emergency that should be treated in intensive care, including administration of intravenous phosphate.

Patients with AN have a lower heart rate, abnormal autonomic nervous system regulation of the heart, lower systolic blood pressure at peak exercise compared with controls, and regional wall motion abnormalities on echocardiography or radionuclide ventriculography, often in the absence of shortness of breath, palpitations, or chest pain. Deficiencies of magnesium, phosphorus, thiamine, and selenium can weaken cardiac muscular contraction. Ipecac ingestion may lead to a reversible weakening of the cardiac muscle. Causes of heart failure associated with AN are listed in Table 4.3.

Arrhythmia

Protein–calorie malnutrition causes electrical changes in the heart, abnormal cardiac pacing, and changes in cardiac repolarisation resulting in prolongation of the QT interval, and ST/T wave abnormalities. Blood pressure is decreased, heart rate is low, and there may be changes in the autonomic function of the heart manifested by increased variability in heart rate and cardiac depolarisation.

Death in AN can be caused by arrhythmia associated with prolonged repolarisation of the ventricles. Drugs prescribed as psychopharmacotherapy or for self-harm include tricyclic antidepressants, major tranquilisers, prokinetic agents, erythromycin, and antihistamines, all of which can prolong the QT interval of the electrocardiogram and predispose to arrhythmias and torsade de pointes.

Table 4.3 Causes of heart failure in AN

Cause	Evidence	Characteristics	Treatment tips
Phosphate deficiency	Good	Sudden onset Serum phosphorus may drop rapidly	Stop feeding Oral and intravenous phosphate
Ipecac toxicity	Good	The toxicity of ipecac varies greatly between patients	Usually reversible with discontinuance
Protein–calorie malnutrition	Good	Slow in onset	Refeed Include adequate protein in feeding
Magnesium deficiency	Good	Rare, even with severe hypomagnesaemia	Intravenous magnesium
Selenium deficiency	Good	Rare Usually in chronic AN	Treat with oral and intravenous selenium
Thyrotoxicosis	Good	May be difficult to diagnose in AN because the symptoms of both are similar Measure TSH	Treat the hyperthyroidism and consider beta blocker
Alcohol	Good	Alcohol is cardiotoxic	Abstinence Thiamine
Thiamine deficiency	Good	Usually presents as Wernicke's encephalopathy, rarely as heart failure (wet beriberi)	Routinely supplement all patients with thiamine during refeeding
Hypoglycaemia	Poor	Hypoglycaemia usually results from insufficient liver glycogen	Intravenous glucose to prevent hypoglycaemia while refeeding
Autonomic dysfunction	Poor	Usually reverses within 3–10 days of refeeding in hospital	Consider using metoprolol to treat arrhythmias

Abbreviations: AN, anorexia nervosa; TSH, thyroid-stimulating hormone.

Why do patients often develop complications after treatment begins who never had them before? Nutritional recovery causes many of the complications. One such change is the rapid decrease in heart rate variability (the change in it – not the amount of it) that occurs when refeeding is done quickly. This stage of treatment may occur again and again if relapse or only partial recovery occurs.

Atherosclerosis

Patients with AN are usually amenorrhoeic, under a great stress, have high low-density lipoprotein and low high-density lipoprotein cholesterol as well as apolipoprotein protein abnormalities, and those who have been in psychiatric inpatient of residential care usually smoke cigarettes. All of these factors increase the risk of atherosclerosis. There have been some reports of significant atherosclerotic lesions in autopsies of patients who died with AN. However, a comparison of carotid arteries of patients with anorexia and controls showed no difference in intimal thickness.

Patients with AN frequently have chest pain. Often they have more than one type at the same time. The causes of chest pain in AN include chest wall pain, reflux esophagitis, oesophageal spasm, chest pain owing to abdominal bloating, Boerhaave's syndrome, functional causes, and typical and atypical angina. Palpitations may be perceived as a chest pain. About 20% of patients interviewed in one study were found to have pain consistent with typical or atypical angina.

Bacterial Endocarditis

Endocarditis is made more likely in AN by mitral valve prolapse, dental caries, and polymorphonuclear leukocytic dysfunction related to magnesium deficiency, zinc deficiency, and severe protein–calorie malnutrition. However, it is rare.

Drug Overdose Treatment – Cardiovascular Considerations

A drug overdose in AN should be managed as in other patients. Be aware of the following:

> The patient is likely to have ingested a variety of pills over the years. They may have access to their old pills as well as pills from their family, and over-the-counter weight loss preparations that contain stimulants like ephedrine.
>
> Self-injurious behaviour is common in hospitalised patients. Patients with AN may split staff and family, steal, and be untruthful. Patients may undo their intravenous catheter or central total parenteral nutrition line; drain the fluid out of lines (risking air embolism); remove, drain, and reinsert their feeding tube; and cut themselves or overdose in hospital.

Do not give intravenous sugar until you give 100 milligrams of thiamine intravenously. Wernicke's encephalopathy can be precipitated by administering intravenous dextrose that rapidly depletes thiamine or if there is a deficiency of phosphate or magnesium that are required for thiamine to function in humans.

These malnourished patients often have no liver glycogen and are therefore prone to hypoglycaemia if intravenous feeding is stopped.

The serum creatinine is usually at the lower limit of normal or below normal because of reduced muscle mass. A normal serum creatinine means the patient is in renal failure. Deficiencies of vitamins and minerals often exist with normal laboratory tests. Low levels of minerals and vitamins occur during hospitalisation are rarely evident on laboratory tests at admission.

An increase in the QTc interval indicates a change of cardiac conductivity. Drugs, magnesium, phosphorus, and potassium should be checked as causes. Prolongation of the QTc interval, which predisposes to arrhythmias, is lower in young women (450 msec) than in middle-aged males.

Gastric hypomotility and oesophageal reflux are very common. Pills may remain in in the stomach for long periods of time. This may limit absorption. There is an increased chance of aspiration.

Hypotension

Blood pressure should be measured lying and then standing using a small-sized cuff appropriate for arm circumference. The lying or sitting blood pressure is usually in the range of 90/70 mm Hg with a heart rate of forty-five to sixty beats per minute. This does not cause symptoms unless it is associated with volume depletion.

Normally, if the patient stands up quickly after lying for a minute or two there will be a brief decrease in blood pressure for up to five to ten seconds with an increase in heart rate by five or ten beats per minutes. If there is volume depletion (dehydration) or autonomic dysfunction, the blood pressure will remain low longer or the heart rate will not increase. A low jugular venous pressure confirms volume depletion, but because vascular responsiveness is usually maintained the jugular venous pressure is often low until volume depletion is marked. Postural hypotension can occur without volume depletion owing to impaired vascular and autonomic responsiveness. Hypothermia, which commonly occurs in AN, can also cause hypotension and decreased vascular responsiveness. Medications can decrease the responsiveness of the vasculature and the heart.

Heart Rate Variability

The heart rate is usually low in AN – in the range of forty-five to sixty beats per minute. However, particularly if the patient is an athlete, the heart rate may be as low as thirty beats per minute. As long as there are no symptoms, this does not increase mortality or morbidity.

Changes in cardiac conduction or heart rate variability may be a sign of autonomic dysfunction and increase the likelihood of arrhythmia. It is the rapid normalisation of heart rate variability the is most likely the cause of this increased risk. Heart sounds are normal in AN. They may be louder owing to the thin chest wall. Mitral valve prolapse, which occurs in about seventeen per cent of healthy young women, is even more common in AN; it worsens as the heart muscle thins as malnutrition worsens and improves as malnutrition improves. As a consequence, midsystolic clicks may be heard, increase in number, be heard with a midsystolic murmur, and eventually disappear as the mitral valve prolapse worsens, leaving the holosystolic murmur of mitral regurgitation. This is usually reversible after weight restoration, although this recovery occurs over a year or two. Mitral valve prolapse is best heard with the patient standing and performing the Valsalva manoeuvre.

The Electrocardiogram

Most patients with AN have a normal electrocardiogram, apart from bradycardia. The following may occur: first-degree heart block, ectopic atrial rhythms, nodal escape, ventricular premature complexes, ST depression, and U waves. Most of these abnormalities normalise within two weeks of correcting deficiencies and feeding. No treatment of arrhythmia is indicated except those indicated by the normal cardiological guidelines.

For clinically important arrhythmias, cardiac monitoring until the abnormality resolves (usually within seventy-two hours) and oral metoprolol between 25 and 100 mg daily should be considered.

The QTc interval (the QT interval corrected for heart rate) is usually prolonged with weight loss. It will commonly be in the range of 350–400 msec in young females. Prolonged QTc is one risk factor for arrhythmia, but arrhythmias may occur without a prolonged QTc. It is likely the relative prolongation of the QTc interval that occurs with weight loss, mineral deficiencies, or drugs is a predisposing factor to arrhythmias.

A QTc interval of longer than 550 msec raises concern for arrhythmias in normal adults. However, we recommend that causes of QT prolongation be sought and treated if the QTc is more than 450 msec or there is an increase of 60 msec beyond the baseline.

Abnormalities of T waves, pacemaker, rhythmicity, and other changes may occur so that the electrocardiogram may seem to be bizarre. In the absence of symptoms, volume or mineral deficiencies, or causative medications, this is likely due to malnutrition alone. An episode of collapse should include investigation of arrhythmia. Remember that hypoglycaemia can cause arrhythmia.

Differential Diagnosis

Heart valve abnormalities can be caused by the use of weight loss medications like D-fenfluramine or L-fenfluramine and phentermine. An echocardiogram should be performed to exclude valvular dysfunction in this setting. Hyperthyroidism can worsen symptoms of an ED as well as predispose to arrhythmia. In the differential diagnosis of AN, Addison's disease, which may cause hyperkalaemia and hyponatremia, low blood pressure, and postural hypotension, should be considered. Repeated doses of ipecac may cause a cardiomyopathy.

Implications for Health Care Professionals

- Cardiac arrhythmia is the most common medical cause of death from AN.
- Heart function is usually within normal limits in AN.
- In low weight AN, the heart wall is usually thinned and the mitral valve changes shape and may leak causing clicks or murmur.
- One measure of the electrical recovery of the conduction system of the heart is the QTc interval reported on the electrocardiogram. In AN the QTc is often prolonged and this increases the chance of arrhythmia and sudden death.
- Heart failure can occur if the serum phosphorus decreases to less than-one half the lower limit of normal. Contact the physician if the serum phosphorus is decreasing. If it decrease below normal, it is critical.
- Monitor the heart rate and blood pressure lying and then standing. The effect of medications, dehydration, and AN may only be demonstrated by the change when standing up.
- Variability of heart rate that is not caused by standing, exercise, or anxiety may be due to dysfunction of the autonomic nervous system, which increases the chance of arrhythmias.

Patient Information

- Report chest pain, palpitations, dizziness, or collapse to your nurse or doctor because these may be symptoms of heart dysfunction caused by the ED.
- The cardiac complications of AN are reversible.

Gastrointestinal

Case

A patient says he believes he has sprue because he feels better when he avoids eating gluten-containing food

Salivary Glands

Enlargement of the parotid and submandibular glands is common in both AN and BN. It may be the only clue to the diagnosis on physical examination. Salivary gland enlargement (parotid and submandibular) can occur to a slight degree owing to protein–calorie malnutrition alone without binging and purging, but is more likely to occur and is more marked with vomiting.

Purging can cause salivary gland hypertrophy by increasing salivary fluid pressure behind the swollen papilla, where fluid empties into the mouth. The glands also enlarge because of marked variability in autonomic nervous function. The glands are controlled by the autonomic nervous system. When there is little stress, the parasympathetic nervous system causes the glands to release saliva – but with stress salivary release stops, causing enlargement of the glands.

Parotid and salivary gland hypertrophy usually resolve after successful treatment of the ED, although this improvement can take several months. Warming turns on parasympathetic (relaxation) tone and results in much more rapid decrease in salivary gland size.

Warming can be applied to the body by use of an infrared sauna once a day for ten to twenty minutes at or above thirty degrees centigrade or by using an electric warming pad on medium heat for one hour three times a day anywhere in the body. This increases the parasympathetic tone of the autonomic nervous system and result in a decreased size of the salivary glands usually within two weeks.

If the parotids are painful owing to enlargement, applying warming as described plus warming over the parotid in combination with mouth irrigation using saline and lemon as mouth wash may rapidly decrease parotid size. Lemon increases salivary flow, but it is acidic and can cause tooth pain. If it causes pain, lemon should not be used.

Rarely, unilateral tender swelling of a parotid gland occurs. This is usually because the patient always sleeps on one side of their body and that side (the dependent side) is more swollen. However, acute suppurative parotitis owing to infection of the parotid usually caused by *Staphylococcus aureus* should be considered. In acute suppurative parotitis, there may be a small amount of white fluid at Stensen's duct where the parotid opens into the mouth next to the second molar. This occurs if the patient is not adequately hydrated and mouth hygiene is poor.

Hyperamylasaemia, owing to release to the enzyme amylase from the salivary glands, occurs after purging. Serum amylase is also made up of amylase from the pancreas, the urogenital epithelium, and small bowel mucosa. Measure serum lipase, which comes only from the pancreas, to exclude pancreatitis. Alternatively, the tissue of origin of the increased amylase can be determined by measuring amylase isoenzymes.

Oesophagus

Repeated vomiting can cause abnormal gastric peristalsis, decreased lower oesophageal sphincter tone, oesophageal reflux, hematemesis (vomiting blood), esophagitis, and even oesophageal rupture (Boerhaave's syndrome). Boerhaave's syndrome is a catastrophic manifestation requiring immediate emergency medical and surgical intervention. Rarely, patients will survive oesophageal rupture without surgery.

Chronic sequelae of recurrent vomiting are oesophageal strictures and Barrett's oesophagus. Barrett's oesophagus occurs when the normal epithelium of the oesophagus is replaced by squamous epithelium, like that of the skin. Barrett's oesophagus can transition to cancer of the oesophagus – so endoscopic follow-up is mandatory.

Mallory-Weiss tears may lead to marked gastrointestinal bleeding. Mallory-Weiss tears occur at the junction of the stomach and the oesophagus, and are caused by the physical trauma of vomiting.

Lesser degrees of oesophageal dysfunction are seen with malnutrition alone. If bisphosphonates are used to treat osteoporosis, care must be taken to monitor for the associated esophagitis and oesophageal stricture.

Stomach

Decreased and impaired motility of the stomach are common. This can result in gastric stasis, early satiety, and predispose to oesophageal reflux. Acute gastric dilatation and rupture have been described in BN during bingeing and in AN during refeeding. The rapid onset of nausea, vomiting, or abdominal pain suggest gastric distension. This can, of course, be due to disorders unrelated to EDs, like gastric torsion or adhesions. Rarely, gastric rupture occurs, which causes severe pain, sepsis, and shock, and requires urgent surgical intervention.

Ball of Hair in the Stomach (Bezoar)

A gastric bezoar is a foreign body that forms and remains in the stomach. If a patient with trichotillomania swallows enough of the hair that they have pulled, a ball of hair can develop in the stomach. A bezoar has often been present for some time before diagnosis because symptoms are not specific. A CT scan of the abdomen is the preferred initial investigation for bezoar because it is sensitive, although not specific. Neither the abdominal radiograph or ultrasound examination is not sensitive for the diagnosis of gastric bezoar. If the CT scan is suggestive, an endoscopy is needed confirm the diagnosis.

Small and Large Bowel

Superior mesenteric artery syndrome presents in very low weight patients as bloating and epigastric abdominal pain that occurs soon after eating and is increased with meal volume. The diagnosis is often missed because patients with an ED usually have abdominal symptoms and they often refuse to eat much.

Look for a history of the pain or discomfort that begins during or shortly after eating accompanied by abdominal bloating in the upper abdomen. The diagnosis is confirmed by demonstrating a narrowed third part of the duodenum with proximal dilatation of the bowel on imaging. This can be seen on ultrasound examination or a CT scan, but if the radiologist has not seen it before they may fail to make the diagnosis. It may be easier for the radiologist to identify the syndrome after eating when the obstruction is more apparent. For treatment, enteral feeding is usually required because regular meals worsen the pain caused by the partial bowel obstruction.

Patients with an ED often have slow and abnormal peristalsis. This can result in postprandial bloating, increased intestinal gas, constipation, faecal impaction, and paradoxical diarrhoea. Laxative abuse can cause or exacerbate symptoms, because the chronic use of stimulant laxatives may result in the loss of normal peristaltic function.

Laxative abusers usually complain of episodes of diarrhoea alternating with periods of constipation. The underlying problem in paradoxical or overflow diarrhoea is constipation. The small hard stools act like logs blocking a river. Like the river, the pressure behind builds up until diarrhoea overflows intermittently, and then the constipation returns until the pressure builds up again.

Cathartic colon can be severe, but rarely necessitates colonic resection. Chronic, recurrent use of laxatives may result in gastrointestinal bleeding, ranging from occult to frank blood loss. Laxative abuse is a cause of nail clubbing. This may reverse if the laxatives are stopped.

Celiac disease or inflammatory bowel disease may coexist with AN, but are not caused by AN. Celiac disease has become common owing to the use of genetically modified grains and the large size of pellets – both increasing the likelihood of allergy to gluten. Celiac disease can result in failure of weight gain because of malabsorption or because of the markedly limited diet the patient must follow. Patients should be tested for antigliadin antibodies before a gluten-free diet is started. They should see a dietitian and become aware of suppliers of gluten-free food; many foods and condiments contain gluten.

Rectal prolapse, faecal impaction, and faecal incontinence can occur in chronic AN owing to weakness of the muscles of the pelvic floor. Rectal prolapse is common in chronic AN. It can cause pain, incomplete defecation, and obstruction. Early intervention may prevent the need for surgery, which is often unsuccessful. Early intervention includes weight restoration, stool softeners, increased fluid intake, prokinetic agents, and exercises to strengthen pelvic and rectal muscles. Many patients who have rectal prolapse have a lack of weight gain owing to an altered diet, abnormal function, chronic anxiety, marital discord, and continued disagreement with physicians, psychologists, bowel therapists, and naturopaths. Team discussions may improve the patient's outcome.

Liver and Gallbladder

The liver and gallbladder are usually normal and unaffected by the ED. A fatty liver can occur with severe protein malnutrition; gallbladder contraction may be slow and cholesterol-containing gallstones are more common after recurrent weight loss owing to supersaturation of the bile with cholesterol.

Pancreas

The pancreas is rarely abnormal. There is no need to have the patient ingest pancreatic enzymes. Type 1 diabetes mellitus often coexists with AN and BN. Acute pancreatitis can develop in BN and the purging form of AN, usually owing to excess alcohol ingestion or biliary tract disease. If signs or symptoms of pancreatitis, such as abdominal pain, nausea, or vomiting are observed, measurement of serum amylase as well as serum amylase isoenzymes or serum lipase and an abdominal ultrasound examination help make the diagnosis. Serum amylase isoenzymes and serum lipase are measured to exclude other sources of increased serum amylase, such as the parotid glands, small bowel, or urogenital organs. However, the abdominal pain is often not investigated because abdominal symptoms are so common in EDs. If pancreatitis is diagnosed, treatment includes admission to the hospital, bowel rest, nasogastric suction, and intravenous fluid replacement.

Digestion

Digestion is normal unless the patient uses laxatives, in which case rapid transit of food may slightly decrease the absorption of calories. Exogenous thyroid or hyperthyroidism can lead to malabsorption. Vitamin B_{12} or folate deficiencies can result in atrophy of the villi of the bowel and malabsorption. Other diseases like inflammatory bowel disease and celiac disease can cause rapid weight loss in a previous weight stable patient.

Frequency of Complications

Usual: decreased gastric and intestinal motility with postprandial bloating, and constipation, salivary gland enlargement involving both the parotid and submandibular glands, absence of liver glycogen.
Common: paradoxical diarrhoea, Mallory-Weiss tear, rectal prolapse.
Uncommon: esophagitis, fatty liver, superior mesenteric artery syndrome.
Rare: peptic ulcer, oesophageal stricture, Barrett's oesophagus, Boerhaave's syndrome, oesophageal rupture, gastric bezoar.

Implications for Health Care Professionals

- Patients with an ED usually have lots of abdominal complaints, and they are more likely to have another disease as a complication of their ED or in addition to it. There you must take a history and do a physical. If the patient has new or worsened symptoms, consider diseases like gastric bezoar, superior mesenteric artery syndrome, pancreatitis, and rectal prolapse.
- Abdominal bloating, intestinal gas, and excessive fullness after eating are very common and should improve with regular meals and snacks, adequate but not excessive fluid intake, fibre, and prokinetic agents if required.
- The patient's ability to absorb foods and the ability of their liver or pancreas to function in digestion is normal. They do not require bile or pancreatic supplements.

Patient Explanation

- You can expect to have some bloating, cramps, and irregularity of bowel movements because your bowel is weak. However, this will improve as your weight and eating habits improve.
- You may require medication to help your bowel return to normal. Your physician may prescribe this. If you use the medications prescribed to you, your bowels will recover faster.
- AN does not cause permanent damage to your bowel or digestive system, but the persistent use of laxatives may.

Endocrine

Case

A hospitalised female patient with an ED complains of painful enlarged breasts and lactation (galactorrhoea). She wants to know the cause – and tells you she cannot be pregnant.

Hypothalamic/Pituitary

Changes in the function of the hypothalamus and pituitary glands are secondary to weight loss. Follicle-stimulating hormone and luteinising hormone (LH) may decrease to prepubertal levels, resulting in amenorrhea in females. There may be some decrease in antidiuretic hormone, resulting in partial diabetes insipidus. Dopamine antagonists like olanzapine and meclopramide cause an increase in prolactin, which may cause decreased libido, breast engorgement, and lactation. Growth hormone is increased in AN, whereas insulin-like growth factor-I levels are low. All of these changes reverse with feeding, so they should not be treated, other than discontinuing or decreasing medications that cause side effects that are intolerable.

Thyroid

As an adaptation to starvation, the metabolic rate is reduced by decreasing circulating active thyroid hormones (thyroxine and triiodothyronine), increasing inactive thyroid hormone (reverse triiodothyronine), while keeping the regulatory hormone from the pituitary (thyroid-stimulating hormone) within the normal range. This lowering of the thermostat is called the sick euthyroid syndrome. Normally, thyroid-stimulating hormone is increased when there is a decrease in active thyroid hormone (hypothyroidism). This is a physiological adaptation to malnutrition; it is not hypothyroidism and should not be treated.

Hyperthyroidism can occur during the course of AN, BN, or binge ED. If it does, it will exacerbate the symptoms and may be difficult to recognise because symptoms overlap.

Adrenal

Hypercortisolaemia occurs in AN. Despite the elevated serum cortisol, adrenocorticotropic hormone that regulates it is normal and there is a decreased response of adrenocorticotropic hormone to its regulatory hormone, corticotrophin releasing factor.

Plasma cortisol and adrenocorticotropic hormone levels in bulimics are usually normal. Nonsuppression on the dexamethasone test occurs in some bulimic patients that may be confounded by comorbid depression or other comorbid disease.

Ovary

Amenorrhea occurs in AN, but it is secondary to hypothalamic/pituitary dysfunction and decreased conversion of hormones by the diminished fat mass, leading to low circulating levels of pituitary gonadotropins. Even with amenorrhea, ovulation may still take place.

Contraception must still be used to protect against pregnancy, despite amenorrhea. Menstrual disturbance often precedes severe weight loss and may persist for many months after weight is regained. Other factors that may stop normal menstrual function include psychosocial stressors, a disturbance of oestrogen metabolism, and a fault in oestrogen feedback to the hypothalamus.

Pelvic ultrasound examination can be used to help determine whether a physiologically normal weight has been attained in the absence of menses. Pelvic ultrasound examination can assess whether ovarian follicles are being formed. Ovarian follicles indicate that a physiological body weight has been reached and normal endocrine function is possible.

The likelihood of a normal pregnancy is less in patients who conceive before they have fully recovered from their illness. Low birth weight and a higher incidence of spontaneous abortion, congenital malformations, prematurity, and perinatal mortality, together with poor parenting, have been reported. Induction of pregnancy by methods such as pulsatile LH-releasing hormone is not medically or psychologically advisable. Reproductive function after recovery, however, is usually normal.

Menstrual abnormalities are also seen in normal weight patients with BN, although less frequently than in AN. In BN, a pattern of irregular menses is more common than amenorrhea. A decreased number of LH secretory spikes and abnormal LH responses to gonadotropin-releasing hormones have been reported in some patients with BN.

Breast

In AN, breast size diminishes in adults, and does not progress in prepubertal females. Breast engorgement and lactation often occur when medications are used that increase serum prolactin, like prokinetic agents.

Temperature Regulation

Patients with AN are less aware of hypothermia and hyperthermia and are less able to regulate body temperature. Hypothermia is common, and fever in the face of infection is reduced.

Other Hormones

Leptin is reduced owing to and in proportion to the reduction in adipose tissue mass. Grehlin may be elevated in AN but normalises with weight restoration. Peroxisome proliferator-activated receptor is normal.

Hypoglycaemia

Hypoglycaemia in AN is common. It occurs after eating – not when fasting. It is most common after an increase in caloric intake, usually during the first week or two of refeeding. If the patient's diet is not consistent, so that it increases and decreases in caloric content, intermittent hypoglycaemia will recur.

In normal subjects, after ingesting a meal there is an increase in serum glucose. This increase is followed by the secretion of insulin from the pancreas to move glucose into the cells where it is needed. Next, to prevent hypoglycaemia (the blood glucose dropping too low), glucagon is secreted from the pancreas. Glucagon causes glucose to be released into the blood from the liver. The liver glucose comes from the breakdown of glycogen stores in the liver. Glycogen is a complex sugar.

However, in AN, the liver glycogen stores are reduced or absent. Thus, no sugar is released from the liver to prevent hypoglycaemia caused by insulin secreted in AN when liver glycogen is low. Low blood sugar, or hypoglycaemia, presents after meals as headache, confusion, impaired consciousness, arrhythmia, seizure, or death. Some patients have no symptoms with hypoglycaemia or ascribe it to the ill effects of eating food.

To rule out hypoglycaemia occur during, refeeding one should measure blood sugar at thirty minutes to two hours after meals, and during the night or when symptoms occur. A blood glucose level of less than 2.5 mmol/l is diagnostic of hypoglycaemia.

Using a finger prick test for glucose is convenient and should be encouraged. However, the error in finger prick glucose is about twenty per cent, and even less accurate for blood sugar of less than 3 mmol/l. Use the finger prick test and the patient's response to ingestion of fast-acting sugar (e.g., orange juice) to confirm the diagnosis. If the finger prick test is around 3 mmol/l or less and symptoms are ameliorated within five minutes of ingesting orange juice, the diagnosis is confirmed.

Alternatively, a glucagon test can be performed. In the fasting state, blood glucose in measured before, ten minutes after, and twenty minutes after the intravenous administration of one milligram of glucagon. A normal response is elevation of glucose of more than 7 mmol/l or an increase of at least 2 mmol/l to greater than 6.5 mmol/l.

If you suspect or have confirmed hypoglycaemia, measuring blood glucose during the night is particularly important because the patient is unlikely to be aware of nocturnal hypoglycaemia. Nocturnal hypoglycaemia may present as sweating, nightmares, palpitations, seizure, or morning headache. If hypoglycaemia has occurred during the night, the body will have corrected the blood sugar by gluconeogenesis by the morning. The morning blood sugar may be normal or even high because of the marked response of the body to hypoglycaemia. Thus, a normal or high morning blood sugar does not exclude the possibility of nocturnal hypoglycaemia. Nocturnal hypoglycaemia is common in patients who eat relatively more at night or binge and purge at night.

Treatment of Postprandial Hypoglycaemia

(1) Treat hypoglycaemia every time it occurs with the ingestion of quickly absorbed carbohydrate like orange juice.

(2) Prevent acute attacks with a constant infusion of intravenous dextrose at a rate sufficient to maintain the blood sugar at greater than 5 mmol/l and/or by meals eaten every four hours, including during the night. The meals must not contain simple sugars and be formulated individually by a dietitian. A 100-mg dose of intravenous or intramuscular thiamine must be administered before the intravenous glucose. Otherwise, Wernicke's encephalopathy may be precipitated by the intravenous glucose. Then, 100 mg of thiamine should be given orally for the next ten days.

(3) Replete the stores of glycogen in the liver and maintain them at normal levels by achieving a normal weight.

Frequency of Complications

Usual: Amenorrhea, infertility, hypothermia, reduction in breast tissue, decrease in libido, hypoglycaemia.

Common: Ovulation and fertility are present despite amenorrhea, sick euthyroid syndrome, hyperprolactinemia owing to medications

Rare: Partial diabetes insipidus, exacerbation of AN by concurrent thyroid dysfunction or thyroid pills.

Implications for Health Care Professionals

- Loss of menstruation does not mean that the patient is not ovulating. Patients may still be ovulating and become pregnant. They must use birth control if they are sexually active.
- The oral contraceptive pill is an ineffective treatment of osteoporosis in AN

- A loss of breast size concomitant with weight loss is normal in the post pubertal female. This reverses with weight recovery. In the prepubertal female with AN, breast development will be halted.

Patient Explanation

- If having no periods is bothersome to you, your doctor can prescribe the oral contraceptive pill.
- Even though you are not menstruating, you may still be ovulating and could get pregnant. You must use birth control if you are sexually active.
- A decrease in breast size (or, if you have not gone through puberty yet, a halt in breast development) is normal in AN. With recovery, breast development will resume.

Kidney

Case

A patient with low weight AN had a kidney test that was better than normal (creatinine). Now it is higher but normal. She asks you whether this means anything.

Kidney Function

Reduced fluid intake and concentrating ability of the kidney may result in urinary frequency and nocturia, decreased urine volume, and predisposition to renal stones (increased urinary ketones also predisposes to renal stones). The serum creatinine should be lower than the normal range because creatinine is proportional to muscle mass and their muscle mass is low. However, creatinine clearance is adjusted for body mass and is a good measure of renal function.

Patients with AN often decrease fluid intake because they have noticed it increases their weight. This leads to chronic dehydration (volume depletion) and reduced renal function. Alternatively. they may believe that large volumes of water are healthy and drink ten litres or more of water a day. An excessive intake of fluid washes out the kidney's ability to concentrate urine. This leads to dehydration if the fluid intake is decreased. This is because the kidney cannot concentrate urine. If the psychological need continues despite explaining the importance of normalising water intake the diagnosis of psychogenic polydipsia should be used. This diagnosis may have to be distinguished from diabetes insipidus or partial diabetes insipidus, which are rare. Diabetes insipidus is due to a decreased amount or action of antidiuretic hormone. A nephrology consultation should be requested if this is questioned.

Renal insufficiency can be caused by vomiting and laxative misuse. Prolonged purging and/or diuretic or laxative abuse can cause dehydration that activates a homeostatic mechanism to prevent dehydration. The renin–angiotensin–aldosterone system reduces urine output and is usually overly effective – resulting in oedema formation. If a patient attempts to decrease their diuretics or laxatives, they usually develop swelling of their ankles. This triggers severe anxiety and consequently the diuretics or laxative are begun again, and often at a higher dose. This self-perpetuating cycle can be extremely difficult to interrupt.

Volume repletion with normal saline will prevent oedema formation if given before refeeding. As an outpatient, Oxo cubes, high-salt miso soup, or other high salt fluids taken three times a day can be used until volume is normalised (dehydration is controlled) or until there is no hypotension on blood pressure testing and normalisation of jugular venous pressure.

The patient must believe that fluid retention is temporary and that it will resolve if purging behaviours are stopped. Dependent oedema should be treated by reassurance; it will disappear without treatment in a week or two. Bed rest and below-the-knee antiembolic stockings may be used to temporarily reduce dependent oedema. If marked fluid retention (e.g., more than six kilograms) threatens compliance, drug therapy may be necessary. Spironolactone, which is a weak physiologic aldosterone antagonist, can be given in doses between 50 and 200 mg a day to be tapered over two weeks. Alternatively, an angiotensin-converting enzyme inhibitor may be used . However, the risk of hyperkalaemia and renal insufficiency limit its usefulness in AN.

With malnutrition, the muscles of the pelvis are weakened. Rectal prolapse may occur and cause high intra-abdominal pressures, which impair bladder function. Autonomic dysfunction causes abnormal contraction of the bowel and bladder and neurogenic bladder dysfunction may occur. These can lead to urinary retention, stress incontinence, and lower urinary tract infections.

Frequency of Complications

Usual: Nocturia, frequency.

Common: Mild azotaemia (usually owing to volume depletion).

Uncommon: Psychogenic polydipsia, urinary incontinence, neurogenic bladder.

Rare: Renal stones,

Implications for Health Care Professionals

- Nocturia is common and is related to malnutrition and decreased urinary concentrating ability. It disappears with feeding.
- Correct volume depletion to prevent oedema before you stop laxatives or diuretics.

Patient Information

- Passing urine at night is common in AN. It is due to a decrease in the ability of your kidney to concentrate urine. This resolves with weight recovery.
- It is important to drink enough fluid, but not too much. Drinking too much fluid can hurt your kidneys. Discuss the volume of fluid you should be drinking with your doctor or the dietician.

Bones and Joints

Case

A patient with AN saw her endocrinologist, who wanted to start her on special bone-forming medications to treat her osteoporosis. She asks you for your opinion.

Bone

Decreased bone mass (osteoporosis or osteopenia, which is decreased bone mass to a lesser degree than osteoporosis) is almost always present in AN. Bone loss increases with time and with the severity of malnutrition. Inadequate diet, low circulating oestrogens, high serum cortisol, laxative misuse, low serum vitamin D_3, an abnormal gut microbiota, autonomic dysfunction, and disturbed acid–base balance contribute to osteoporosis. Osteoporosis is more likely in those with abnormal gut bacteria. The abnormal gut bacteria (microbiota) cause or are caused by autonomic dysfunction of the nervous system. Direct treatment of gut bacteria for the treatment of osteoporosis is not proven.

The epiphyses are the part of bones are where linear growth occurs. Their ability to permit growth stops in the late teenage years. If AN occurs before the patient's growth is complete and recovery does not occur before the epiphyses close, their full adult height will never be reached. Many patients are brought for treatment in their late teens too late to grow past an early adolescent height.

As osteoporosis increases, the risk of fracture is increases. At first, stress fractures will occur in the weight-bearing bones of the feet, lower limbs, and pelvis. Stress fractures are similar to the tiny cracks in cement one sees in the sidewalk. They are very painful but do not change the overall symmetry of the bone involved. Later vertebral fractures occur, decreasing height and often resulting in chronic back pain that can continue until death.

Osteoporosis is decreased bone mass. Osteomalacia is a decrease in bone mineral density. Rarely, patients with AN have osteomalacia, so it is usually not considered as a possibility. The most common cause of osteomalacia in AN is low serum vitamin D. This most often occurs in patients who avoid the sun, as in those whose body must be entirely covered from head to toe at all times. Osteomalacia can be distinguished from osteoporosis in that it causes muscle weakness, bone soreness, and rib fractures. Osteoporosis usually causes fractures in thoracic and lumbar spine, wrist, and hip.

The treatment for osteopenia and osteoporosis includes:

- Normalising total body fat. This is the most important and reliable method of improving bone density in AN.
- Using low bone density as motivation for weight gain.
- Optimising diet including, calcium, phosphorus, and magnesium intake. normalising exercise. Inadequate exercise decreases bone mass, but excess exercise reduces the likelihood of weight gain and increases the likelihood of stress fractures and exercise addiction.
- A serum vitamin D_3 level should be measured in all patients with osteoporosis or osteopenia. Start vitamin D_3 supplementation at 2000 I.U. daily and increase until the serum vitamin D is within normal range.

There is no good evidence that exogenous oestrogen (the birth control pill) is useful in the treatment of osteopenia or osteoporosis in AN. However, exogenous oestrogen always decreases their motivation to gain weight as part of the treatment. Bisphosphonates can be tried with marked or symptomatic osteoporosis, especially if there is no improvement with the other treatments listed.

Joints

In adolescents, and sometimes in adults, pain that comes from the hip is felt in (referred to) the knee. Most joint-related abnormalities are due to osteoporosis or overexercise. Overexercise often leads to stress fractures that cause extremely tender points on bones. Concomitant osteomalacia can causes hip pain and bone pain.

Vitamin A toxicity can cause bone swelling and bone and joint aching. Scurvy causes bone disease, including bleeding until the surface of the bone (subperiosteal hematoma), which is very tender.

Meralgia paresthetica causes pain or an odd sensation in the area of the hip and thigh that is often wrongly considered to be due to hip disease. It is due to compression of the lateral femoral cutaneous nerve in low weight patients owing to a lack of fatty tissue to cushion the nerve.

Frequency of Complications

Usual: Decreased linear growth in adolescents, reduced bone mass.

Common: Osteoporosis, stress fracture.

Uncommon: Pelvic fracture, vertebral fracture.

Rare: Osteomalacia causing muscle weakness, bone soreness, and rib fractures (usually owing to aversion of sunlight in AN).

Implications for Health Care Professionals

- Osteoporosis and osteopenia should be used to motivate the patient to gain weight. Weight gain is the single most important and reliable method of increasing bone density in AN.
- Do not suggest the use of exogenous oestrogen as a treatment for osteoporosis in AN. Although it may have benefit in some patients, it always decreases the patient's focus on weight gain and reduces their likelihood of recovery.
- Normalise the diet and ensure adequate vitamin D_3, calcium, magnesium, and phosphorus intake.
- If the patient has an aversion to sunlight, consider osteomalacia.
- If severe osteoporosis exists and the patient cannot gain weight, consider a trial of bisphosphonates.

Patient Explanation

- AN causes weaker bones (osteoporosis). However, if your weight returns to a healthy level, your bones can return to normal.
- Osteoporosis increases over time with continued malnutrition, but improves with weight restoration.
- Your bones continue to build and remodel all your life until death. The lengthening of your bones stops after the teen years.
- It is important to take vitamin D, calcium, and other medications as prescribed, but there is no substitute for weight recovery.
- Osteoporosis leads to bone fractures, inability to exercise, and often chronic pain.
- Children and adolescents must weight restore if their bones have not stopped lengthening or they will not reach their adult height.

Blood

Case

A depressed patient with an ED, who is a health care professional, has a sudden large drop in their haemoglobin.

Haemoglobin

Haemoglobin is usually slightly below normal levels in AN owing to an anaemia of chronic disease. Anaemia of chronic disease is a secondary sideroblastic anaemia that results from impaired transfer of iron to red blood cells. Anaemia in AN can also be due to deficiencies of iron, vitamin B_{12}, folic acid, and rarely, copper or vitamin C. Rarely, bone marrow failure, resulting from drug toxicity or severe malnutrition, causes a severe anaemia. This can be life threatening.

Anaemia can also be caused by self-phlebotomy (the patient bloodletting themselves). Self-phlebotomy should be suspected if the haemoglobin level decreases quickly, if the haemoglobin decreases by more than thirty per cent, if there is no nutrient deficiency, or if the patient has unexplained needle marks. Almost all cases of self-phlebotomy occur in health care workers.

White Blood Cells

The white blood cell count is usually slightly low in AN, secondary to protein–calorie malnutrition. However, the neutrophil count is usually high enough to protect against bacterial infections (greater than 500 cells/mm^3).

Immunity may be abnormal in malnutrition owing to other factors besides the neutrophil. With malnutrition deficiency the neutrophils may not function if the proteins in the blood that are necessary for the immune process (e.g., interleukin-1b, interleukin-6, and tumour necrosis factor-alpha) or minerals (e.g., magnesium, zinc) are deficient.

A megaloblastic anaemia with a decrease in white blood cells can result from deficiencies of vitamin B_{12}, folate, or copper. If bone marrow failure occurs, the neutrophil count may decrease to less than 500 cells/mm^3. In AN, bone marrow failure is usually associated with a greater decrease in haemoglobin than white cells or platelets. The lymphocyte count is usually normal.

An increased eosinophil count of greater than 500 cells/mm^3 occurs in Addison's disease, allergies (including drug allergy), collagen vascular disease, foreign body reaction, and cancer. Addison's disease can mimic AN. If there is an elevated eosinophil count, Addison's disease should be ruled out by testing.

Bleeding

Platelets

The platelet count is usually normal and does not cause bleeding. The platelet count can be low in vitamin B_{12}, folate, or copper deficiency, from drugs or alcohol, or from bone marrow failure.

Coagulopathy

Coagulopathy and trauma must be excluded if excess of unusual bleeding occurs (bleeding does not stop, bleeding occurs with little trauma, there are multiple or unusual locations or bleeding). Vitamin K deficiency, liver failure, and disseminated intravascular coagulation have been reported in AN. Vitamin K is a fat-soluble vitamin formed by bacterial flora in the bowel and the vitamin K dependent coagulation factors (II, VII, IX, and X) are formed in the liver. These are usually unaffected by AN.

Scurvy

Vitamin C deficiency is very unusual in AN, but this author still's at least one case a year. Vitamin C deficiency causes excess bleeding from the gums, under the surface of the bones (under the periosteum) with minor trauma, and most commonly as pin head sized bleeding around hair follicles on the thighs (perifollicular haemorrhages).

Frequency of Complications

Usual: Mild anaemia and leukopenia.

Common: Iron deficiency anaemia, in AN after 10 years, B_{12} deficiency.

Uncommon: Anaemia or leukopenia owing to vitamin B_{12} or folate deficiency, anaemia from self-phlebotomy.

Rare: Anaemia from copper deficiency, bone marrow failure owing to drug toxicity, coagulopathy, bleeding from scurvy.

Implications for Health Care Professionals

- Mild anaemia and leukopenia are common in AN and usually require no treatment other than nutrition and weight restoration.
- Mild leukopenia is not associated with an increased risk of infection.
- Deficiencies and self-phlebotomy may cause marked anaemia.
- The neutrophils may be made inactive owing to deficiencies of immune regulating proteins or minerals.

Patient Information

- A slight lowering of haemoglobin or white blood cells is common in AN. Usually, there are no ill effects – although it is a sign you are unwell.
- Iron deficiency anaemia is common in EDs, especially if the diet is strictly vegetarian or vegan.
- Tell your doctor if you have bleeding, including menstrual bleeding.

Immunity

Case

A patient gets staphylococcal abscesses of her skin whenever she loses weight. When she gains weight she get viral infections.

Although the chance of someone with AN getting a bacterial or fungal infection is the same as others, their body's ability to respond to and recover from bacterial and fungal infections is impaired. Their febrile response to bacterial infection is delayed, as is their inflammatory response to both bacteria and fungi. The cause of this is not clear, although it may relate a decreased ability of their white blood cells to move to the site of infection and be active there, as a result of impaired cytokine production, and sometimes mineral deficiencies. There is increased spontaneous and stimulated levels of proinflammatory cytokines, such as interleukins (interleukin-1b, interleukin-6) and tumour necrosis factor-alpha.

Patients with AN are less likely to get viral infections. Once they weight restore, they get viral infections at the same rate as others.

Cellular Immunity

Cellular-mediated immunity is decreased only with severe malnutrition. Low magnesium also causes white blood cells to be dysfunctional. Zinc deficiency may cause decreased cellular immunity. Vitamin B_{12} and folate deficiencies can cause low white cells counts, rarely to a level (less than 500 cells/mm^3), where infection is more likely.

Antibodies

Antibody production and levels are normal. Therefore, immunisation should be given as usual.

Frequency of Complications

Usual: Slightly low neutrophil count of no significance unless there is an abnormality of cytokines, magnesium, or zinc.

Common: If bacterial infection should occur, it will take longer to cause symptoms such as fever, it will not respond normally to treatment, and there is an increased likelihood of complications. Thus, bacterial pneumonia is more likely to progress to lung abscess and empyema, a fungal skin infection is more likely to extend, osteomyelitis starts with no associated pain or signs of inflammation and grows large, and staphylococcal skin infections will relapse and remit. Weight restoration will improve outcomes.

Uncommon: Decreased cellular response owing to magnesium or zinc deficiency.

Rare: Agranulocytosis associated with bone marrow failure.

Implications for Health Care Professionals

- Viral infections are less frequent in AN. Bacterial infections are no more frequent than in normal weight patients, but if they do occur, there is a delay in symptoms and they respond poorly to treatment.
- There is a decreased febrile response to bacterial infection in AN.

Patient Information

- The immune system usually functions normally in AN. You can receive vaccination as usual and you are no more likely than others to get a viral or bacterial infection.
- If you do get a bacterial or fungal infection (such as pneumonia or a urinary tract infection) you may not develop a fever or other signs or symptoms and the infection may be more severe. You must therefore get treatment early for bacterial or fungal infections.

Chapter 5

Complications of Nutritional Therapy

Study Questions

- How many calories is it possible to "burn" in a day by exercise or non-exercise activity thermogenesis?
- Explain how an accelerometer and a metabolic cart could be used to answer those questions and how you could make use of them in a patient.
- Does the Harris-Benedict Equation correctly estimate caloric need during refeeding? Explain your answer.

Fundamentals of Nutrition

Nutrients can be classified as macronutrients (proteins, fats, and carbohydrates) or micronutrients (vitamins and minerals). Malnutrition is, by definition, a deficiency or excess of a nutrient or macronutrients. A malnourished patient may have a single deficiency (e.g., iron deficiency) or multiple deficiencies (e.g., protein-calorie malnutrition, iron deficiency, and vitamin B_{12} deficiency).

Nutrients are usually ingested as food, absorbed through the gut, transported in the blood, and may be stored in the body (e.g., vitamin B_{12} is stored in the liver). The amount of a particular nutrient that is stored and where it is stored varies greatly. For example, the average length of time that stores last if the intake of these nutrients ceased is nil for zinc (brain zinc), a few months for magnesium, three to five years for vitamin B_{12}, and seventeen years for selenium and vitamin A.

Most clinicians test for the deficiency of a nutrient by measuring its blood level. However, blood levels of nutrients do not reflect what is stored in the body. If the intake of a nutrient decreases to less than its requirement, the stores of that nutrient will gradually be used up. Although the stores become depleted, the serum level usually remains within normal limits. Serum levels of nutrients can also be misleading if the organ in which the nutrient is stored is inflamed (vitamin B_{12} is released into the blood with any inflammation of the liver), if the carrier protein of the nutrient is abnormal (e.g., retinal binding globulin is required to transport vitamin A; Figure 5.1), or if there is a deficiency of the cofactors that are absolutely necessary for the nutrient to function (e.g., thiamine requires magnesium and phosphorus to function; Figure 5.2). Therefore, pathophysiological abnormalities can result from a nutrient even when the serum level of the nutrient is normal.

A balance study tests for a deficiency by comparing input and output of the nutrient. Thus, if a patient is not deficient (e.g., magnesium) all of that nutrient given to the patient in an infusion will be excreted. Conversely, if the nutrient was deficient, some of the nutrient given in the infusion would be retained the body for use or storage.

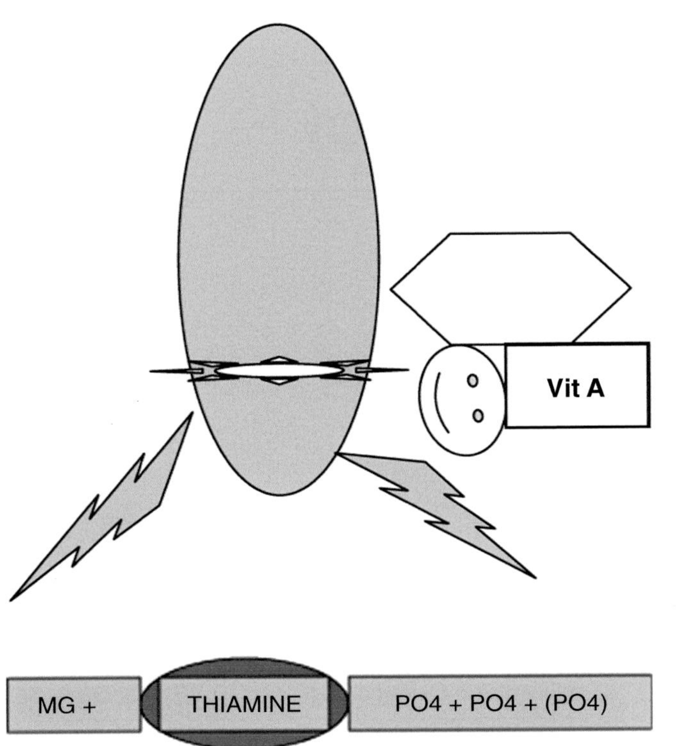

Figure 5.1 Vitamin A requires a specific carrier protein to function.

Figure 5.2 Thiamine is inactive without phosphorus and magnesium.

The sum of the intake versus the use and excretion of a nutrient determines the amount of a nutrient in the body. This is analogous to predicting the level of water in a bath. The level is determined by the rate water pours into the bath from the tap on the one hand, and the rate that water leaves the bath on the other. Even if the drain is completely plugged, the bath will only gradually fill. Like the bath analogy, if the intake of a nutrient is a below normal, the amount in the body will gradually change until it reaches steady state. In the case of nutrient this may take days, weeks, months, or even years.

Another reason that a screening blood test may be normal in patients with severe malnutrition is the reduced rate of nutrient use in malnourished patients. Malnourished patients have a reduced metabolic rate and a greatly reduced rate of tissue formation and turnover. Importantly, once refeeding begins, the rate of nutrient use increases dramatically, associated with an increased metabolic rate within a few days, even without weight gain. Nutrient demands increase even more with weight restoration. It is difficult for patients to understand how the metabolic rate could increase over a few days when the decrease in metabolic rate associated with plateauing during dieting takes six to twelve weeks. If they do not understand this process, they may resist increasing their calorie intake during refeeding and prolong their recovery.

Thus, the blood levels of vitamins and minerals are a poor measure of their stores in the body. The body adapts to a decreased nutrient intake by lowering the metabolic rate, reducing the use of nutrients, and by forming a new equilibrium between serum levels and stores. An increase in the number of calories eaten rapidly increases the metabolic

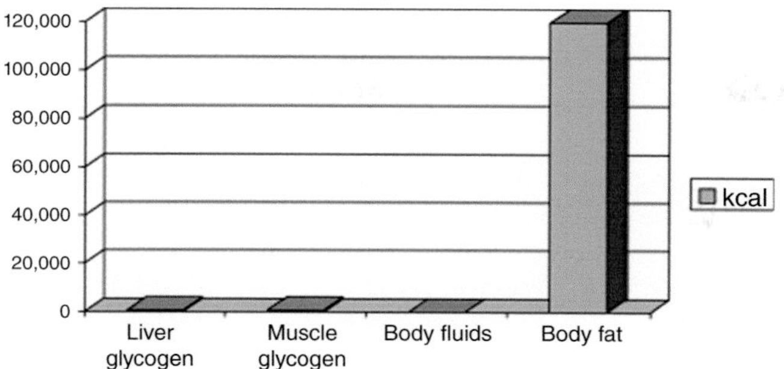

Figure 5.3 Where is energy stored in the body?

rate and the rate of use of other nutrients, uncovering deficiencies and leading to the refeeding syndrome, morbidity, and sometimes death.

Patients may better understand this concept using the analogous situation of a lot on which a house is to be built. The lot is empty, but then filled with all types of materials in preparation for the building of the house. One can only judge whether the materials are sufficient, however, when the building is underway and suddenly the builder runs out of nails, or wood, or windows. It is the building stage the uncovers a lack of building supplies.

Energy

The energy needed for the body to function is provided by nutrition. More than ninety per cent of the body's available energy is stored in adipose tissue. The rest of the energy is provided by the small amount of carbohydrate (glycogen) in the liver and muscle (Figure 5.3). The patient's fear of body fat is magnified exponentially by increases in body fat. Using skinfold callipers to demonstrate the thickness of body fat and the thickness of the goal body fat is often pleasantly surprising to the patient.

Protein–Energy Malnutrition

When the body takes in less energy than it requires, stored energy is used. All tissues of the body needs glucose for energy. As the blood glucose level decreases, insulin falls, glucagon rises, and later cortisol and catecholamines increase. With starvation, carbohydrate (glycogen) stores are used first, followed by adipose tissue (fat), and then protein (amino acids). When fat is broken down, ketone bodies increase in the blood causing a mild acidemia. Usually this acidemia is mild and accompanied by a decrease in serum bicarbonate of just a few millimoles per litre. The brain is the only organ that can switch to ketone bodies for energy after a day or so of starvation. In about two per cent of patients, starvation ketosis results in a severe and progressive acidaemia. Ketone bodies are osmotically active and carry water from the body through the kidney, along with minerals. This process results in dehydration. Protein loss causes a gradual wasting of the muscles of the body, including the respiratory muscles and the heart.

Most patients with anorexia nervosa (AN), even those who are severe malnourished have a normal serum albumen (marasmus). Some, however, develop low albumen, a fatty liver, and the bloated picture known as kwashiorkor, which results from a low intake of energy and protein in the diet. A high-protein diet should contain 1.5 rather than 0.7–1.0 grams of protein per kilogram of body weight per day. A dietitian should prescribe the diet. Details of important deficiency states are listed in Table 5.1.

Table 5.1 Nutritional deficiencies

Deficiency	Store	Symptoms and signs	Features of deficiency	How to monitor and treat	How long to treat
Magnesium	Weeks to months	Muscle cramps Weakness (proximal myopathy) Fatigue of the focus of the eyes Impaired short-term memory	Although a low level always indicates deficiency, most deficiencies occur in the face of normal serum magnesium. A magnesium load test is required if the test is normal and symptoms of muscle cramping, muscle weakness, fatigue of the focus of the eye or impaired memory are present.	The preferred route is intravenous magnesium (see Orders). Magnesium can be given intramuscularly, but is painful. Oral magnesium is very poorly absorbed, but can be used in addition to other routes or as prophylaxis.	Usually requires 5–10 intravenous treatments. Until symptoms disappear and serum levels remain normal. The gold standard of adequate repletion is magnesium load test at the end of treatment.
Phosphorus	Days to weeks	Usually presents as the sudden onset of congestive heart failure	Independent of body stores, the level of phosphorus decreases immediately after eating and increase quickly with ingestion of phosphorus. A decreasing level or a subnormal level is an indicator of increased risk of the medical consequences of phosphate deficiency (e.g., congestive heart failure, Wernicke–Korsakoff syndrome) and must be treated.	Daily serum phosphorus during rapid weight gain ($\geq$1 kg/wk or more). Then three times a week for 3 weeks then once a week, if gaining 0.5 kg a week or more.	Provide prophylaxis for as long as, and whenever, rapid weight gain occurs plus another 2 weeks.

Potassium	Days to a week	Muscle weakness (proximal myopathy) Palpitations	Serum level is fairly proportional to total body stores. Serum potassium is spuriously increased in acidaemia and tissue injury (haemolysis in the blood tube will increase the level); and decreased with alkalosis. Serum potassium usually decreases because of potassium loss in vomitus, but can decrease because of a lack of renal reabsorption owing to magnesium deficiency. If the kidney is wasting more than 5 mmol/l of potassium on a single urine sample, in the face of low serum potassium, suspect magnesium deficiency as the cause.	Measure serum potassium daily during the first week of rapid weight gain, then three times a week if weight gain continues at greater than 1.0 kg/wk. Later, if weight gain continues at 0.5 kg, measure once a week.	Give 20 mmol/l of potassium chloride three times a day gradually decreased to 20 mmol/l once a day over 2–3 weeks. Continue as long as weight is gained at greater than 0.5 kg a week. decrease or stop potassium supplementation with renal dysfunction or low urine output.
Calcium	Months to years	Muscle cramping, carpopedal spasm (latent tetany), palpitations, dysrhythmias, seizures	The level of the free (unbound) calcium in the blood is normally carefully controlled by serum parathormone. Low levels of serum calcium in AN indicate the protein that carries calcium is low, but the free level is not (measure serum free calcium, which	Measure serum calcium at the beginning of refeeding to rule out a primary calcium abnormality. Then do not repeat its measurement unless muscle cramping or carpopedal spasm occurs.	If the ionised calcium is low, and the cause is not total body magnesium deficiency, the treatment and treatment duration depend on the underlying cause.

Table 5.1 *(cont.)*

Deficiency	Store	Symptoms and signs	Features of deficiency	How to monitor and treat	How long to treat
			will be normal) or there is a total body magnesium deficiency (this causes low calcium by reducing the parathormone effect and secretion). The treatment of the latter is magnesium deficiency treatment.		
Thiamine	Days to weeks	Wernicke's encephalopathy (confusion, nystagmus or ophthalmoplegia, and ataxia) Much less commonly, neuropathy or congestive heart failure	Deficiency can by precipitated by intravenous glucose.	Avoid intravenous glucose. Monitor for and treat hypophosphataemia and hypomagnesaemia. If Wernicke's encephalopathy is present, give thiamine 100 mg intravenously and intramuscularly immediately and 100 mg intramuscularly daily for 10 days and correct hypophosphataemia and hypomagnesaemia.	Treat acute Wernicke's encephalopathy with 20 days of thiamine and correction of phosphorus and magnesium deficiencies.
Iron	Months to years	Tiredness, pica (abnormal food cravings, the most common being for ice and cold beverages), and anaemia	Serum ferritin is often low in AN owing to very low oral intake.	Supplementation can cause constipation, black stools and upset stomach. Start supplementation with concurrent anaemia or after initial refeeding is progressing well. Give ferrous sulphate, gluconate, or fumarate	The iron supplementation should be continued for 6 months without anaemia and for 12 months with associated anaemia.

				300 mg once a day, gradually increasing to three times a day if tolerated.	
Folic acid	Weeks	Tiredness Anaemia	Serum folic acid changes quickly with diet, so RBC folate should be ordered instead. RBC folate is usually normal in AN. If the RBC folate is low, this is usually due to a decreased intake of green leafy vegetables. Folate is quickly used in cell production (particularly red blood cells), so it should be supplemented when iron or B_{12} are given for anaemia, irrespective of its level. A high RBC folate is usually due to vitamin ingestion that contains folate.	Folic acid orally in a dose of 5 mg.	The folic acid supplementation should be continued for 1 month, but longer if the haemoglobin is increasing or if the diet is low in green leafy vegetables.
Vitamin B_{12}	3–5 years	Tiredness and fatigue Yellowish skin and sclera Anaemia Dementia Loss of normal gait and vibration and joint position sense Peripheral neuropathy	Vitamin B_{12} is only absorbed in the terminal ileum and only if bound to intrinsic factor produced in the stomach. It is stored in the liver and is necessary for cell division through the body. A low level is usually due to dietary deficiency, but about 3% to 9% of the time it is	Vitamin B_{12} by injection, 1000 μg daily for 3 days and then 100 μg monthly for 3–5 years. If the Schilling's test is normal, still give the injections for 6 months and then use oral B_{12} tablets 50 μg a day. Do not give tablets with vitamin C or iron at the same time as vitamin B_{12} tablets because	Continue for 3–5 years. If there is an abnormal Schilling's test, there may have to be lifelong supplementation. However, usually the abnormal Schilling's test is due to vitamin B_{12} or folate deficiency, causing intestinal cell atrophy. So

Table 5.1 *(cont.)*

Deficiency	Store	Symptoms and signs	Features of deficiency	How to monitor and treat	How long to treat
			due to malabsorption. The Schilling's test is necessary to determine whether malabsorption is the cause of the B_{12} deficiency.	these agents decrease its absorption.	the Schilling's test can be rechecked in a few years and parenteral supplementation stopped.
Vitamin K	A week to weeks	Bleeding or bruising that is delayed after trauma	The bacteria in the bowel manufacture vitamin K. The absorbed vitamin K is necessary for the production of all the coagulation factors except factor VIII.	Treatment is by the injection of a solution of 10 mg of vitamin K or, if absorption is certain and there is no vitamin K, deficiency is assessed indirectly by measurement of the coagulation by ordering an INR. Vitamin K deficiency causes a raised INR. A level of 10 g/dl is to be expected in AN owing to the anaemia of chronic disease that is usually a secondary sideroblastic anaemia that needs no treatment other than treatment of the AN. A level lower than this may be due to low iron, low vitamin B_{12}, low folate, self-phlebotomy, marrow failure, low copper or drug toxicity. A haematologist should	One injection or 5 days of oral acute bleeding, give 10 mg vitamin K orally for 5 days.

				inspect the blood film (RBC morphology); ferritin, vitamin B_{12} and RBC folate should be ordered with a haemoglobin of less than 10 g/l. A haematological consultation should be obtained if the cause is not clear.	
Vitamin A	17 years	Night blindness Bitot's spots (appearance is like little bits of meringue on the sclera) Collapse of the globe of the eye	Measuring serum vitamin A levels can assess a vitamin A deficiency. This test is expensive and need only be ordered if a deficiency is suspected. Vitamin A is bound in the blood to retinal-binding globulin (RBG) that is made in the liver. Patients who have severe protein deficiency (low albumin) or liver impairment may have a low serum vitamin A owing to a low RBG level, with no deficiency of vitamin A. Conversely, when the RBG gets very low, vitamin A cannot be delivered to the tissues, even with treatment, and tissue damage owing vitamin A deficiency will occur	Treatment is oral vitamin A, 5000–50 000 I.U. per day depending on the seriousness of the deficiency. If too much vitamin A is ingested toxicity results leading to many systemic symptoms, including bone aches and those resulting from increased intracranial pressure	Continue vitamin A for a few months; during that time assess and increase vitamin A in diet if possible, and start a multivitamin that contains vitamin A

Table 5.1 *(cont.)*

Deficiency	Store	Symptoms and signs	Features of deficiency	How to monitor and treat	How long to treat
Pyridoxine	Months to years.	Peripheral neuropathy Anaemia	Deficiency is rare in AN	Treat deficiency with 100 mg pyridoxine.	Continue oral pyridoxine for 3 months.
Zinc	Weeks to months	Weight loss, impaired or abnormal taste (dysgeusia) Dry peeling skin (especially on the palms and soles) Decreased cellular immune function	Zinc is mainly found in milk products and seafood and is bound to fibre in the diet. Copper and zinc compete for the same absorptive pathway. If copper is taken in large quantities for long periods of time, zinc deficiency may develop, and vice versa. Zinc intake in AN, especially with quasi-vegetarian diets, is very low. Oestrogen increases urine loss of zinc. In AN, zinc deficiency usually presents as dry skin and decreased taste sensation. Serum zinc can be measured but does not reflect zinc stores unless it is low. Zinc is bound to albumin and zinc-binding globulin, so patients with low serum protein will seem to have low serum zinc despite normal free serum zinc. Zinc deficiency can be	Give 14–28 mg/d of elemental zinc (zinc gluconate 100–200 mg/d) for 2 months.	Routine treatment with zinc in AN for 2 months. Treat deficiency state for 6 months.

			measured by taste testing (e.g., the Accusens T Test); however, we have not found this sensitive or specific to zinc deficiency.		
Riboflavin		Angular stomatitis		Prevent by giving a daily multivitamin. Treatment of the deficiency is with a multi-B vitamin for 1 month.	Give for 1 month and then multivitamin for a year.
Copper		Megaloblastic anaemia, thrombocytopenia, and leukopenia, together or individually	Copper deficiency is rare in AN. The bone marrow shows changes indistinguishable from those seen in folate or vitamin B_{12} deficiency. Suspect copper deficiency with anaemia, thrombocytopenia, or leukopenia that is progressive, undiagnosed, and seems to be megaloblastic. Taking 400 mg or more of zinc gluconate a day for more than 4 months can cause copper deficiency.	Treat with oral copper, a few milligrams a day of elemental copper as the sulphate form.	Give for 3 months.
Selenium	17 years	Proximal myopathy, cardiomyopathy	Selenium is found in fruits and vegetables. It is low in the soil in New Zealand, parts of Canada, and China. Vegetables marketed come	Treat a symptomatic deficiency with intravenous selenium, as administered to patients receiving total parenteral nutrition. Treat a	

Table 5.1 *(cont.)*

Deficiency	Store	Symptoms and signs	Features of deficiency	How to monitor and treat	How long to treat
			from around the world, so low selenium ingestion is rare. Selenium is necessary for the metabolic function of the mitochondria. A deficiency is usually caused by malabsorption coupled with low intake. Deficiency is very rare in AN. Suspect selenium deficiency if a severe undiagnosed myopathy develops in a patient with chronic severe AN. A low serum level is not diagnostic of a clinical deficiency.	low serum level with an oral vitamin containing selenium.	

Abbreviations: AN, anorexia nervosa; INR, international normalised ratio; RBS, red blood cells.

Fluid, Electrolytes, and Minerals

Serum creatinine is proportional to body muscle. The amount of muscle is decreased in AN – so the serum creatinine is low, too. Thus, serum creatinine may be in the normal range, even when there is marked kidney dysfunction in AN.

Dehydration is the most common cause of kidney dysfunction. Vomiting can cause loss of stomach acid, fluid, and potassium and result in decreased serum potassium (termed hypokalaemia hypochloraemia [metabolic alkalosis]). This condition can usually be treated with oral fluid and potassium replacement (see Medical Complications). However, potassium must not be given orally or intravenously until the patient has passed urine to avoid dangerously high serum potassium.

Low serum magnesium (hypomagnesaemia) is common in patients with an eating disorder (ED). Muscle weakness in the large muscles, cramping of the leg muscles at night, difficulty maintaining visual accommodation, and impaired short-term memory are typical signs and symptoms of total body magnesium deficiency. Magnesium deficiency also impairs the ability of the kidney to retain potassium. This deficiency should be suspected if low potassium does not correct with supplementation. In this case, magnesium must be given to correct a low serum potassium. Magnesium deficiency can also cause hypocalcaemia and hypophosphataemia.

Hypophosphataemia usually occurs during refeeding owing to the huge uptake and need for phosphate by cells during feeding – leading to the refeeding syndrome. Hypophosphataemia can occur very rapidly, resulting in heart failure and death within days of feeding. Phosphate blood levels must be watched carefully (daily) during refeeding – particularly in the first ten days. The higher the caloric content of the diet, the faster the weight gain, and the more likely hypophosphataemia is to occur. Daily serum levels of phosphate should remain almost constant. If serum levels begin to decrease, extra oral phosphate should be given. Should the levels decrease quickly, death can occur. Phosphate falls after meals in all of us as it is moved into the cell with glucose and insula, so blood work must be done in a fasting state because the serum phosphate changes temporarily after eating.

Patients with an ED can have bizarre diets that result in unusual deficiencies, such as copper. Copper deficiency can also be caused by excessive intake of zinc for more than a few months. Zinc and copper share the same pathway of absorption in the proximal bowel – too much zinc means too little copper gets through.

Concurrent causes of malabsorption like gut resection or celiac disease can produce deficiencies earlier than usual or of unusual types, such vitamin B_{12}, vitamin A, vitamin C, and selenium.

Are All Patients with EDs Malnourished?

People who binge and purge can have nutrient deficiencies even though their weight loss may be less extreme. In addition to the ED diagnosis itself, the duration of the ED, the recent course of the ED, medications, eating and purging behaviours, food intake, intake of fibre (binds some nutrients), where there food was grown (certain soils are deficient in some nutrients), and comorbidities (e.g., gastrointestinal disease, hyperthyroidism) all affect a patient's nutritional tatus.

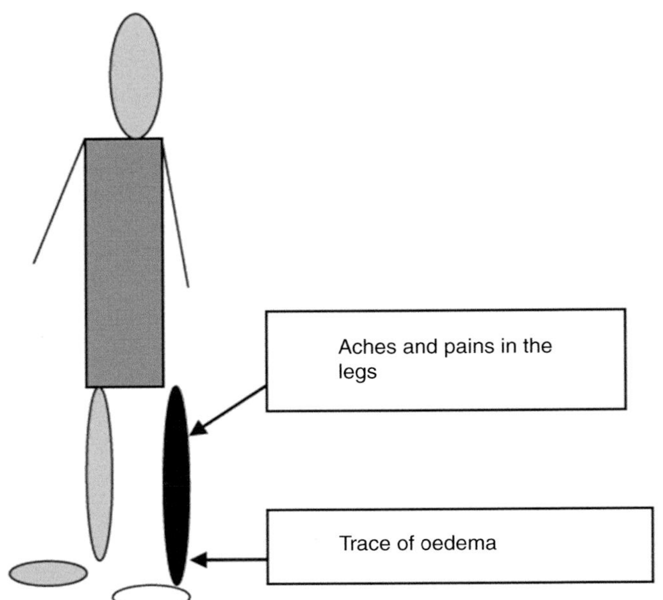

Figure 5.4 The historical meaning of the refeeding syndrome.

What Is the Refeeding Syndrome?

What Does "The Refeeding Syndrome" Mean?

The term refeeding syndrome has two meanings. The historical meaning (Figure 5.4), is the combination of symptoms and signs that usually occur in malnourished patients during refeeding. These symptoms are dependent oedema and aches and pains, especially in the legs. The dependent oedema, often referred to as refeeding oedema, occurs even if the patient was not dehydrated and has a normal serum albumen at the beginning of treatment. It is due to the decreased renal function and low metabolic rate that accompanies malnutrition. The oedema is much greater if dehydration or low albumen is present.

Figure 5.5 illustrates the current meaning of the refeeding syndrome, that is, the symptoms and signs of the deficiencies that develop as a consequence of feeding. The following sections explain this potentially lethal consequence of feeding and how to prevent and treat it. Table 5.2 outlines a protocol to prevent the refeeding syndrome.

What Causes the Refeeding Syndrome?

The malnourished body has inadequate nutrients to complete the process of rebuilding the body. Also, the amount of each nutrient that is stored in the body is highly variable. Typically, stores of vitamin K last a couple of weeks, vitamin B_{12} last a few years, and selenium a couple of decades. In addition to these deficiencies, AN is associated with bizarre eating habits. Patients may ingest only watermelon or oranges for months. Feeding provides carbohydrate, some fat, protein, and small amounts of vitamins

Table 5.2 How to prevent the refeeding syndrome

Dietitian to order diet (start with low-calorie diet (e.g., 800 kcal/d) and increase gradually)
Laboratory
Haemoglobin, white blood cell count, platelet estimation, serum sodium, potassium, chloride, bicarbonate, blood urea nitrogen, creatinine, creatinine phosphokinase, aspartate transaminase, alkaline phosphatase, magnesium, calcium, phosphorus, ferritin, vitamin B_{12}, red blood cell folate, zinc, international normalised ratio (INR), thyroid-stimulating hormone
Electrocardiogram, urinalysis, routine bloodwork, and microscopy
Routine repeat blood work
Potassium, phosphorus, and magnesium daily for 7 days and then every Monday, Wednesday, and Friday.
Routine supplements
Potassium chloride (pills, effervescent or liquid) 24 mmol three times a day for 21 days
Sodium phosphate solution 5 ml (550 mg of phosphorus) three times a day for 21 days
Multivitamin, two tablets a day for 2 months and then 1 tablet a day
Thiamine 100 mg a day for 5 days
Zinc gluconate 100 mg daily for 2 months
Black strap molasses 15 ml three times a day for 2 months for magnesium
Intravenous rehydration
Administer intravenous normal saline (0.9% NaCl solution) at 100–150 ml per hour until intravascular volume is normalised
Note: The refeeding syndrome usually occurs in the first ten days of marked increase in caloric intake.

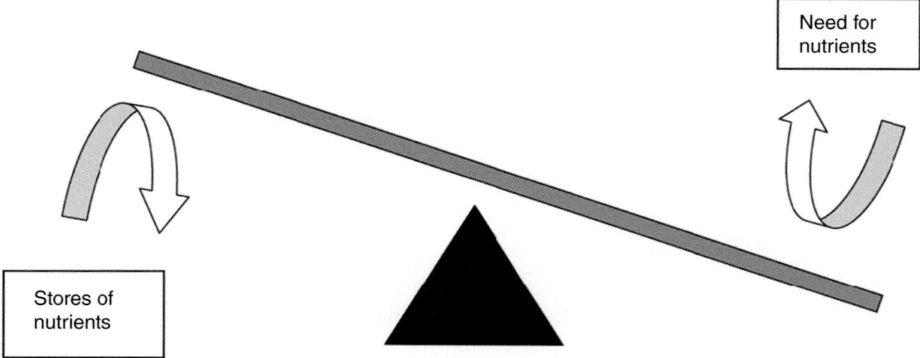

Figure 5.5 The current meaning of the refeeding syndrome.

and minerals to the body. The stores maintained by the body and the body's tendency toward equilibrium explain why the initial blood work is usually normal in AN, and why many deficiencies develop during refeeding. The symptoms that occur during refeeding result from the deficiencies that occur. The nutrient deficiencies that are the most common causes of early death – potassium, magnesium, and phosphate – must be monitored and treated.

The medical symptoms and signs of AN and, although less serious, of other EDs, are part of the illness; thus, it is more appropriate to think of them as medical manifestations rather than merely complications. Although the ED usually starts in adolescence, the course is often prolonged, and people may be ill for many years, and the majority of severely ill patients with AN are in early or mid-adult life. Hence, AN is a matter of concern for adult physicians as well as for paediatricians and adolescent medicine specialists. Figure 3.1 provides a mnemonic that is useful for remembering the physical signs of EDs.

Manifestations result from starvation or from the behaviours adopted to induce it. They are not indicative of underlying pathology. The inexperienced clinician who undertakes unnecessary investigations to exclude all possible causes for each abnormal finding is doing the patient a disservice by delaying appropriate treatment and decreasing the likelihood of the recovery by demonstrating their ignorance. Rather, all clinicians should be aware of the wide range of physical abnormalities that are commonly found in patients with AN (Table 5.3). Many of these abnormalities, such as decreased serum concentrations of gonadotropins and steroid sex hormones, alterations to the peripheral metabolism of thyroid hormone, and increased circulating concentrations of cortisol and growth hormone, are best regarded as physiological adaptations to the state of starvation and do not require treatment.

However, some medical complications are not only clinically important, but also life threatening; these complications require special attention. The body mass index, body fat, and initial laboratory measurements are not, by themselves, reliable indicators of the risk of complications. The risk of serious complications is increased when the patient gains weight, increases the frequency or amount of purging by any method, starts to binge, or is noncompliant with medications or starts self-medicating or using recreational medications. Life-threatening complications, especially vitamin and minerals deficiencies, are most often precipitated by rapid refeeding.

Implications for Health Care Professionals

- Blood tests are poor indicators of nutritional deficiencies.
- Some deficiencies are due to lack or excess of a carrier protein or another vitamin or mineral and can, therefore, occur even when there is adequate supplementation.

Patient Information

- Your body has stores of vitamins and minerals that last between one day and seventeen years. In addition, your food intake has been different for some time and you may run out of nutrients like vitamins or minerals when you increase your intake.
- How nutrient deficiencies develop. Nutritional deficiencies can be understood by using the analogy of a university student's struggle with money. At the beginning of their studies, a student has money in the bank, money in their pocket, a car, an apartment, and money for activities. As time goes by, the money in the bank goes first. They still have money in their pocket, although perhaps their activities are limited. Next, they may have to sell the car. Gradually, their possessions diminish

Table 5.3 Summary of possible medical abnormalities in patients with eating disorders

Metabolic	Hypothermia and dehydration Electrolyte disturbances (hypokalaemia, hypomagnesaemia, hypocalcaemia, and hypophosphataemia) Hypercholesterolaemia Hypoglycaemia and increased liver enzymes
Cardiovascular	Hypotension, bradycardia, prolonged corrected QT interval, arrhythmia Decreased myocardial wall thickness Attenuated response to exercise Pericardial effusion
Neurological	Pseudoatrophy of the brain Abnormal electroencephalograph and seizures Peripheral neuropathy Compression neuropathy Impaired autonomic function
Haematological	Anaemia: usually normochromic, normocytic Leukopenia, thrombocytopenia Iron deficiency anaemia Megaloblastic anaemia owing to folate, vitamin B_{12} or rarely copper deficiency Hypocellular bone marrow Scurvy
Renal	Prerenal azotaemia Partial diabetes insipidus Acute and chronic renal failure
Endocrine	Low gonadotropins, oestrogens, testosterone Sick euthyroid syndrome Increased cortisol and positive dexamethasone suppression test Increased growth hormone
Musculoskeletal	Cramps, tetany, muscle weakness Osteopenia, stress fractures
Gastroenterological	Swollen salivary glands, dental caries and erosion of enamel (with vomiting) Superior mesenteric artery syndrome Delayed gastric emptying, severe constipation, and bowel obstruction Irritable bowel syndrome, melanosis coli (from laxative misuse)
Immunological	Decreased interleukin-1 and tumour necrosis factor-alpha leading to more severe bacterial infections (staphylococcal lung abscess and tuberculosis)

until finally they are left with little money in their pocket, little or none in the bank, no car, no outings, and a shared room at the dorm. The money in this analogy represents a nutrient – money in the bank is the stored nutrient, pocket money is the serum level of the nutrient, and the money spent on activities is the physiological process for which the nutrient is required. Notice that the tissue levels (the bank) started to decrease first and the serum levels were ,normal even when the stores were nearly exhausted. It is essential that health care professionals who treat patients with EDs understand that the serum levels (the pocket change) do not reflect the body stores of the nutrient. Notice also that the organ damage owing to nutrient deficiency (the loss of possessions, car, their own apartment) happen suddenly, at different points along the way.

- Serum levels are usually poor indicators of the amount of a nutrient in the body. Serum levels often decrease late in the course of a deficiency. A measurement of the total amount of a nutrient in the body, if available, is a better indication of nutritional status. Most total body measurements are tissue measurements. However, the amount of a nutrient varies between organs. The hospital may offer a tissue magnesium measure using white blood cells. However, this measure is a poor indicator, because the white blood cell magnesium is not stable and does not correlate with other tissues. For magnesium the gold standard measurement is a bone biopsy, which is not a convenient measure. Organ damage can occur suddenly and without warning symptoms or signs.
- We will give you supplements that are important to take to prevent deficiencies.
- We will measure your blood to see whether you are developing deficiencies.

Chapter 6

Laboratory Testing

Study Question

- *What vitamins or minerals should be supplemented during early refeeding?*

What Tests Should Be Ordered as Part of the Initial Assessment?

- Complete blood count, electrolytes, blood urea nitrogen, creatinine, creatine phosphokinase (CPK) magnesium, phosphorus, calcium, aspartate transaminase (AST), alkaline phosphatase, ferritin, red blood cell folate, vitamin B_{12}, thyroid-stimulating hormone (TSH)
- Electrocardiograph (EKG)
- Urinalysis
- Dual energy x-ray absorptiometry scan for bone density (for anorexia nervosa [AN] only).

What Tests Should Be Reordered During Treatment?

If the caloric or carbohydrate intake is increased enough to result in a weight increase of 0.5–1.0 kg per week (this is typical of refeeding in hospital):

- Creatinine, magnesium, phosphorus, potassium, daily for 7 days from the beginning of refeeding and then every Monday, Wednesday, and Friday for 3 weeks (or until weight remains stable and serum levels of magnesium, phosphorus, and potassium are stable).
    - Blood sugar 30 minutes to 2 hours after meals (especially if the meal is high in calories or sugars) and whenever symptoms suggestive of hypoglycaemia occur.
- EKG. Reorder the EKG if a medication is started that is known to prolong the QT interval and a few days later because the effect on the QT interval may take a few days to develop. Reorder a stat EKG and request a cardiological or internal medicine consultation if the patient has shortness of breath, dizziness, collapse, chest pain brought on by exertion and relieved by rest, the QTc is greater than 450 msec or increased by more than 50 msec, there is an arrhythmia (other than sinus arrhythmia or occasional premature contractions), heart block, or a strain or abnormal pattern on the EKG.

If there is no increase, or a slow increase in caloric or carbohydrate intake so as to cause a weight increase of less than 0.5 kg per week (as is usual in residential treatment and outpatient treatment):

- Magnesium, phosphorus, potassium, one to three times per week from the start of refeeding for 21 days and then once a week (must increase to two to three times a week if the rate of refeeding increases) depending on the rate of weight gain, the premorbid nutritional state, and change in serum levels.
- EKG as above

Diagnostic Tests Commonly Ordered and Their Limitations

(Alphabetical order)

Note: Many of these tests and procedures are unreliable, unavailable, or costly (Table 6.1).

Alkaline Phosphatase

Serum alkaline phosphatase levels are increased with obstruction to the ductal system of the liver or an increased rate of bone formation (e.g., fracture or during the bone repair phase in AN). Alkaline phosphatase is an enzyme found in bone and liver. Even a single small obstruction to the ducts of the liver can cause an increase in the alkaline phosphatase. To determine whether an increase originates in the liver or bone, order a serum gamma glutamyl transaminase (GGT), because gamma glutamyl transaminase is only released by the liver. An elevated gamma glutamyl transaminase means that the alkaline phosphatase increased is due to liver disease.

AST

The serum AST serum level normally remains constant in an individual. AST is released from the liver cells (hepatocytes) when they are damaged. Elevation of AST is caused by liver damage or muscle damage because AST is found in muscle as well. The elevation of AST is influenced by the amount of damage and by the number of the cells that are damaged. The increase in AST is much greater from the same injury to a healthy liver than to a cirrhotic (scarred) liver. To determine whether an elevated AST is due to liver or muscle injury, a serum CPK test can be measured. CPK is specific for muscle, not liver. An elevation of gamma glutamyl transaminase or nucleotidase is specific for liver damage. CPK is often elevated with overexercise, but only remains elevated for a day or two. Showing a patient their elevated CPK after exercise often causes them anxiety because it shows they are breaking down their muscle. Repeating the CPK with and without exercise usually leads to decreased exercise.

Bicarbonate

Serum bicarbonate is usually normal. It is decreased in acidosis, usually owing to starvation ketosis. It is increased by a hypokalaemia metabolic alkalosis owing to dehydration (volume depletion), especially with vomiting. The kidney will retain sodium in exchange for potassium in an attempt to correct the volume depletion, causing the hypokalaemia.

Blood Count

The complete blood count provides measures of the haemoglobin, white blood cells, and platelets. Severe malnutrition usually results in a mild normochromic normocytic

Table 6.1 Diagnostic tests and their limitations

Name	Measures	Primary indication	Limitations	Danger	Cost
Body mass index	Change in weight corrected to height	To measure the success of feeding	Does not measure whether the change in weight is due to a change in fat, muscle, water, constipation, etc.	None	Low
Anthropometrics	Total body fat	To measure the success of feeding	The reliability of the test is very low unless it is performed by an experienced observer.	None	Low
Electrocardiogram	Electrical activity of the heart	Measures QT interval, heart rate, heart rhythm	Only takes a 20-second record. It is unlikely to capture an intermittent problem.	None	Low
Echocardiogram	Size, shape, and contraction of the heart, as well as valve function	Determines the cause of many heart murmurs, the thickness of the muscle of the heart and its contractile function	Does not measure electrical activity and is insensitive to certain heart conditions like mitral valve prolapse.	None	Moderate
Holter monitor	Measures electrical activity of the heart for 24 or 48 hours on one lead.	Helps to determine the cause of palpitations, faints owing to dysrhythmias and the degree of autonomic dysfunction	Does not use all of the standard heart leads, so not all parts of the heart will be assessed. Does not assess the anatomy or physical function of the heart.	None	Moderate
Chest radiograph	The gross anatomy of the chest and upper abdomen	Helps to determine the cause of shortness of breath and the location of a nasogastric tube placed for feeding	Does not measure lung function. Aspiration may not show up on the chest radiograph for up to 24 hours. The nasogastric tube can move after the radiograph is taken.	Low	Low
CT head	Structure of the brain	Differential diagnosis of loss of consciousness or seizures	Does not measure function.	Low	High

Table 6.1 *(cont.)*

Name	Measures	Primary indication	Limitations	Danger	Cost
CT abdomen	Anatomy of the intra-abdominal organs	To rule out the superior mesenteric artery syndrome	Does not look into functional causes or the microanatomy of abdominal complaints.	Low	High
MRI head	Anatomy of the brain	Best current technique to image the anatomy of the brain	Does not look at brain function. Not as available as CT.	Low	Very high
Functional MRI	Anatomy and some functionality of the brain	May be as good as PET for measuring brain function	Unknown.	Low	Very high
PET scan of brain	Function of the brain	To determine functional brain abnormalities	Very expensive and not generally available.	Low	Very high
Gastric emptying by nuclear medicine	The time taken by the stomach to empty	Differential diagnosis of early satiety and upper abdominal pain	Does not show the anatomy of the bowel.	Low	Moderate
Upper gastrointestinal endoscopy	Appearance of the oesophagus, stomach and part-way down the duodenum	Differential diagnosis of dysphagia, odynophagia, early satiety, abdominal pain, and haematochezia	Does not measure the contraction of the bowel or rule out superior mesenteric artery syndrome.	Moderate	High

CT, computed tomography; MRI, magnetic resonance imaging; PET, positron emission tomography.

anaemia. The haemoglobin rarely decrease to less than 10 g/l owing to malnutrition without another complication. A haemoglobin of less than 10 g/l is most often due to dietary-induced iron deficiency, but it may be due to gastrointestinal blood loss, vitamin B_{12} deficiency, folic acid deficiency, copper deficiency, or self-phlebotomy.

Calcium

Serum calcium is usually normal. A low serum calcium is usually caused by low total body magnesium. Total body magnesium is necessary for the body to maintain serum calcium levels. A low total body magnesium reduces the release and effect of parathyroid hormone and thereby causes hypocalcaemia.

It is the free ionised calcium in the blood that is physiologically active. A decreased serum albumen will result in a low serum calcium because most calcium is carried in the blood by protein. Calcium is bound to albumen for transport so there will be less calcium measured. But the physiologically active (free) calcium is normal. So, if the serum calcium is low, measure the serum free calcium as the definitive test of physiologically important serum calcium.

CPK

Serum CPK should be low in AN owing to low muscle mass. CPK comes from inside muscle cells. Elevation of CPK is caused by muscle damage (smooth or striated). CPK may increase dramatically (ten to thirty times normal) after exercise in AN. To document, take a blood sample within one day of the exercise. Showing a patient their elevated CPK after exercise often causes them anxiety because it shows they are breaking down their muscle. Repeating the CPK with and without exercise usually leads to decreased exercise.

Creatinine

The serum creatinine should be below normal in AN because the level of creatinine in the blood is proportional to the total body muscle mass. An increase in serum creatinine in AN, even to within the normal range, usually indicates renal dysfunction owing to dehydration. Examine the patient for dehydration by measuring the jugular venous pressure and the change in blood pressure and heart rate when standing up after lying down for a few minutes. Dehydration must be treated, or the degree of renal dysfunction may increase.

Increased muscle breakdown may result in a transient increase in CPK. The most common cause of renal dysfunction in AN is dehydration (intravascular volume depletion). Other causes are renal stones, infection, medications, and urinary tract obstruction owing to impaired emptying of the bladder caused by constipation, autonomic dysfunction, or pelvic muscle weakness.

Serum Ferritin

Iron deficiency is common in AN. The main dietary source of iron in the Western diet is red meat, which is usually avoided by patients with eating disorders (Eds). Menstruation, if it continues, also causes iron loss. This is usually the case in AN when the birth control pill is prescribed. Iron deficiency results in tiredness largely owing to the associated anaemia. Iron deficiency can effect taste sensation and eating behaviour. The syndrome of pica, which is seen in some patients with iron deficiency, is characterised by unusual cravings like dirt or paint. The commonest form of pica is pagophagia, the craving for ice and very cold liquids. Ask your patient with iron deficiency whether they have developed a craving for ice or very cold liquids. Some patients with iron deficiency will develop spooning of their nails. This sign has the appearance of a drop of water making an imprint in the middle of the nail.

Folic Acid

Green vegetables are the main source of folic acid (folate) in the diet. Folic acid deficiency may be seen when the patient first presents. Deficiency of folate causes a megaloblastic anaemia that accounts for some of the tiredness experienced in folate deficiency. Folate deficiency can be caused by refeeding. This often goes undetected and limits cell growth and division. It also increases the likelihood of birth defects should pregnancy occur.

Always measure the intracellular level of folate, the red blood cell folate (not the serum folate); it is a more stable indicator of folate status. The serum folate measures all forms of folate, not just the active form. Certain nutrient deficiencies interrupt the folate cycle, causing a traffic jam behind this metabolic block. This means there could be a deficiency of active folate with a normal or elevated serum red blood cell folate. Treating a borderline folate-deficient patient with vitamin B_{12} can precipitate folate deficiency, and vice versa. Because of the greater importance of vitamin B_{12} always treat vitamin B_{12} deficiency first with intramuscular vitamin B_{12} and give an oral folate supplement concurrently.

Magnesium

Total body magnesium deficiency is common in AN. Serum magnesium levels are usually normal, even when there is a total body deficiency. Symptoms of magnesium deficiency are muscle cramping (particularly in the legs at night), weakness of the large muscles, loss of visual accommodation while focusing on a close object (reading), and impaired short-term memory. Signs of magnesium deficiency are proximal muscle weakness (e.g., walking upstairs or strength testing of shoulders), Trousseau's sign, Chvostek's sign, and the lateral peroneal nerve tap sign.

More than 99% of magnesium is intracellular. Body stores are usually very low before the serum level drops below normal. A low serum level always indicates deficiency, but a normal level does not exclude a deficiency. Normal serum magnesium with symptoms or signs of hypomagnesemia is an indication for treatment. If in doubt, perform a magnesium load test. A magnesium load test is performed by measuring the amount of magnesium in a 24-hour urine sample starting from the beginning of the infusion where 20 ml of magnesium sulphate in 250 or 500 ml of saline is given intravenously over 3 or 4 hours. This is a balance test. If the patient is deficient, they will retain 30% or more of the magnesium; if they are not deficient, all of the magnesium will be in the urine sample.

Most diuretics and all proton pump inhibitors can cause magnesium loss in the urine. Patients with an ED are commonly given proton pump inhibitors like ranitidine for stomach upset. Remember that this can cause hypomagnesemia.

Spironolactone is a diuretic that decreased magnesium loss in the urine. Magnesium deficiency causes low serum calcium 80% of the time, low serum potassium 30% of the time, and low phosphate 15% of the time.

Oral magnesium supplementation is usually insufficient to treat symptoms of hypomagnesemia and replete body stores of magnesium. However, one form of oral magnesium seems to be as effective as intravenous magnesium – black strap molasse (Black treacle in the UK). Black strap molasses is the product of the initial crush of sugar cane that is not further refined. It has high concentrations of nutrients, including iron and magnesium. The dosage of black strap molasses to treat hypomagnesemia or symptoms of magnesium deficiency that is not immediately life threatening (seizure or arrhythmia owing to hypomagnesemia) is 15 ml of black strap molasses three times a day. This dose should be continued for one month and then it can be reduced gradually to twice and day and then once a day. The duration of this supplementation depends on the degree of total body deficiency.

If the patient has seizures or arrhythmias owing to hypomagnesemia, the usual intravenous or intramuscular protocol should be followed.

Oral black strap molasses can be ingest by itself, in beverages like tea, chai tea, coffee, with foods like apple sauce, or in cooking or baking.

Phosphorus

Phosphorus is abundant in food, easily absorbed from the bowel, and quickly moves into cells along with glucose after meals. The serum phosphorus level often falls slightly below normal after eating because it moves into cells with insulin and glucose. Phosphorus deficiency is life threatening because phosphate is necessary for adenosine triphosphate, cyclic adenosine monophosphate, 2,3-diphosphoglyerol, and many other metabolic processes.

Phosphate deficiency can cause congestive heart failure, organic brain syndrome, rhabdomyolysis, haemolytic anaemia, and dysfunction of all metabolically active organs in the body. The metabolic complications of hypophosphatemia usually begin once the serum phosphate falls to less than one-half of the lower limit of normal in an ill patient, or less than one-third the lower limit of normal in the healthy patient. Serum levels may decrease rapidly in malnutrition. Any decrease in phosphorus must be treated urgently. The variability of the serum phosphate level is confusing. It is critical that the fasting levels of phosphorus be followed daily during early refeeding and gradually less frequently with time. Any decrease in the serum level should be met by increasing phosphate intake (e.g., cow's milk or phosphate tablets) or decreasing caloric intake to keep the levels stable and in the normal range. Waiting for the levels to get to one-half normal is a recipe for disaster!

Potassium

Serum potassium is commonly low in AN and bulimia nervosa. Hypokalaemia is due to vomiting, diuretics, or laxative abuse, or renal loss owing to exchange for sodium in volume depletion. The degree to which the serum potassium is decreased below normal is proportional to the degree of total body deficiency of potassium. Low total body magnesium increases urine loss of potassium about 30% of the time. If this occurs, the serum potassium will not increase despite potassium supplementation. Potassium in doses of 20–60 mEq per day may be required to correct potassium deficiency, depending on the degree of deficiency, ongoing losses, and the rate of weight gain.

Sodium

The serum sodium is usually normal. The most common abnormality of sodium is low serum sodium caused by the body retaining because of dehydration. This occurs because the body gives a greater priority to protecting blood volume than keeping the concentration of sodium normal. Because all the water ingested is retained, it gradually dilutes the concentration of sodium. Treatment is to increase the amount of salt and water to allow the kidney to correct the concentration of sodium.

Serum sodium can be very low if it is caused by psychologically based water intoxication (psychogenic polydipsia) in AN, Addison's disease (where it is usually associated with an increased serum potassium), hypothyroidism, renal failure, and in the face of diuretic use, because diuretics decrease the ability of the kidney to regulate sodium balance.

Thyroid-Stimulating Hormone

Order the thyroid-stimulating hormone (TSH) blood test to screen for thyroid dysfunction. The TSH assay is very reliable and sensitive, and is the best single measure of thyroid function, usually obviating the need for other screening tests. Release of the thyrotropin-releasing hormone from the hypothalamus stimulates the release of TSH from the pituitary gland, which in turn stimulates the thyroid gland itself to release the thyroid hormones, thyroxine and tri-iodothyronine. The TSH level is increased in hypothyroidism as the body attempts to stimulate thyroid hormone production by the thyroid. The TSH level is low if the thyroid is overactive or with the administration of thyroid hormone.

The sick euthyroid syndrome (euthyroid sick syndrome, thyroid allostasis in critical illness, tumours, uraemia and starvation, nonthyroidal illness syndrome, or low tri-iodothyronine low thyroxine syndrome) when the body tries to downregulate thyroid function. In the case of starvation, this helps to prevent further weight loss and death. Sick euthyroid syndrome is common in AN and should not be treated.

Hyperthyroidism and hypothyroidism can occur during the course of any ED. Hypothyroidism that is associated with an increased TSH causes tiredness, weakness, and depression. It is treated with thyroid supplementation. Hyperthyroidism is more difficult to recognise because it presents with worsening of bingeing and purging, weight loss, and many other symptoms. It should be suspected if the clinical course of a patient changes without cause. In hyperthyroidism, the TSH will be low.

> Patients with major depressive disorder may receive a fast-acting thyroid hormone (Cytomel, triiodothyronine) if they are not responding to other medications. Cytomel causes dysregulation of TSH that can last for months or years. During this time TSH and thyroxine should be measured because the TSH is not a reliable indicator of thyroid function.

Urinalysis

The urinalysis is usually normal. Blood in the urine may indicate renal stones. White blood cells in the urine usually indicate infection, which is made more likely with sexual activity, dysfunction of bladder emptying secondary to weakness of the pelvic muscles, autonomic dysfunction of the bladder, rectal prolapse, or medications. Protein in the urine can be elevated by strenuous exercise. Elevated urine protein can also by a sign of renal damage. Urinary abnormalities are more common in patients with rectal prolapse. Patients should be asked whether they suffer from rectal prolapse because they may otherwise be too embarrassed to speak of it.

Vitamin B_{12}

Serum vitamin B_{12} is usually within the normal range in AN. It is low in about 3% of patients. The serum vitamin B_{12} assay may be falsely low, normal, or high owing to measurement error. This is usually due to a faulty measurement kit. Any inflammation of the liver will falsely increase the serum vitamin B_{12} level. A low serum vitamin B_{12} is usually due to decreased intake, but malabsorption can cause vitamin B_{12} deficiency in patients with an ED.

The Schilling test can be ordered to determine whether vitamin B_{12} deficiency is due to the lack of an intrinsic factor in the stomach, disease of the ileum, or decreased intake. A family history or presence of other indications of polyglandular autoimmune syndrome like vitiligo or celiac disease increases the likelihood of pernicious anaemia as the cause of the vitamin B_{12} deficiency.

Zinc

The serum zinc level does not measure total body zinc. Most zinc is intracellular and there is no store of zinc in the brain. Zinc is bound in the blood to zinc-binding globulin and albumen. Zinc status can be assessed by taste sensation, for example, with the Accusens T Test. However, taste testing is cumbersome and unreliable. Zinc deficiency is best diagnosed by a dietary history of low zinc intake (dietary zinc comes mainly from cow's milk products and seafood) combined with symptoms of zinc deficiency: dysgeusia (altered taste sensation), dry skin on the palms and soles, delayed healing of cuts on the skin, or increased skin infection. Zinc deficiency can occur if excess amounts of copper are taken for months. Zinc and copper compete for the same path of absorption so excess copper can decrease zinc absorption.

Procedures

Chest Radiographs

Order a chest radiograph if respiratory symptoms are present, such as shortness of breath, cough, or chest pain. The most common important finding on chest radiograph is pneumonia. Impaired consciousness or the presence of a nasogastric tube increase the likelihood of aspiration pneumonia owing to aspiration of gastric contents. Radiographic changes may take more than 24 hours to become apparent after aspiration, especially if the patient is dehydrated (intravascular volume depleted). Pulmonary venous redistribution may be the only abnormality on a chest radiograph in acute pulmonary oedema owing to phosphate deficiency. Empyema, often in conjunction with undiagnosed pneumonia, requires immediate hospitalisation.

Echocardiogram

The echocardiogram can be used to assess ventricular wall thickness and the cause of a cardiac murmur. In patients with AN, over time the thickness of the heart muscle decreases. With weight restoration, it can recover over a few of years. As the thickness of the heart decreases in size, the chambers of the heart change slightly. resulting in mitral valve dysfunction. Clinically, this begins with clicks (up to ten clicks may be heard) and later a murmur as blood leaks back through the valve that should be closed. The clicks or murmur of mitral valve prolapse are accentuated by the patient performing the Valsalva manoeuvre while standing. The echocardiogram may miss the mitral valve prolapse because it is routinely performed in quiet respiration while lying. A small pericardial effusion (fluid between the heart and the surrounding sac) is commonly detected by echocardiography in AN, it is of no clinical significance.

EKG

The most common finding on EKG is a slow heart rate (bradycardia). This may be normal in those who do aerobic training long term, but may also be due to malnutrition, hypothyroidism, and the sick euthyroid syndrome seen in AN.

An increase in the QT interval beyond 500 msec may increase the risk of death in AN. The time the ventricular muscle needs to recharge electrically and repolarise is called the QT interval. It is adjusted for heart rate to calculate the QTc or corrected QT interval. This correction is used because the time for repolarisation gets longer as the heart rate gets slower and the heart rate can be very slow in AN.

Prolongation of the QTc interval is not a reliable indicator of an increased risk for sudden death in AN. However, quite apart from that, a prolongation of the QTc interval may indicate an increased risk of arrhythmia if it is due to drugs, deficiencies, or intrinsic cardiac disease. Because AN is often accompanied by deficiencies of nutrients and the use of medications that can increase the QTc interval, an increase above baseline of 50 msec or a measure of greater than 500 msec to convey increased risk of arrhythmia. The QT interval can be prolonged by certain medications and medication interactions that involve the cytochrome P450 system. It may be several days before the QTc interval is prolonged after a medication is started.

Holter Monitor and Spectral Analysis

The 24- or 48-hour Holter monitor captures the EKG recording to assess heart rate, heart block, arrhythmias, and changes consistent with ischemia. In AN, the Holter monitor can help to determine the cause of palpitations on history or arrhythmia on examination. Patients should be instructed to continue their normal activities during the Holter recording. Otherwise, they may avoid activity to decrease their chance of having an arrhythmia.

The heart rate increases or decreases in response to body's need for blood flow. This response changes with rest, exercise, or fear, for example. The heart rate is regulated by the autonomic nervous system. The stress or activation of the sympathetic nervous system, increases heart rate. Calming, or activation of the parasympathetic nervous system, decreases the heart rate.

Heart rate variability is a measure of the function of the autonomic nervous system. Increased heart rate variability that is greater than normal variation in autonomic function is abnormal. Increased heart rate variability is often seen in severely malnourished patients with AN. As in other cardiac disease, increased heart rate variability does not increase the risk of arrhythmia. However, rapid change in heart rate variability does increase the risk of arrhythmia. This often occurs when refeeding begins in AN. Spectral analysis measures the heart rate variability using a computer analysis of the EKG recording. If there is rapid change in heart rate variability, there is an increased risk of arrhythmia during refeeding. Thus, it is not the increase in heart rate variability, but rather the rapid change in heart rate variability that increases the risk of arrhythmias. In most cases, this will occur with rapid feeding, either supervised or unsupervised. By analogy, you could say that a car that can go very fast and very slow is not more likely to crash, but one that has a rapid change in speeds is.

Pelvic Ultrasound Examination

Return of menses is a good marker of normal physiology, but not an ideal marker because menses may be delayed for 6 months or longer after a physiologically normal body fat level is reached. Occasionally, menses will occur sporadically. It is possible to order a pelvic ultrasound examination to visualise the ovarian follicles. Ovarian follicles that are 2 cm in diameter or greater indicate normal endocrine function. This means the patient has a physiologically normal body fat. This is particularly important because the goal body mass index and body fat vary by ethnicity, age, sex, and individual.

Upper Gastrointestinal Endoscopy

Upper gastrointestinal endoscopy can be ordered to investigate severe oesophageal reflux, dysphagia, persistent odynophagia, or hematemesis.

Implications for Health Care Professionals

- Deficiencies will develop during the process of feeding.
- Hospital admission laboratory testing: daily for 7 days from the beginning of refeeding and then every Monday, Wednesday, and Friday for 3 weeks.
- Residential and outpatient treatment lab testing: Magnesium, phosphorus, potassium, one to three times a week from the start of refeeding for 21 days and then once a week (must increase to two to three times per week if the rate of refeeding increases), depending on the rate of weight gain, the premorbid nutritional state, and change in serum levels.

Patient Information

- Monitoring of nutritional status with blood tests is needed during treatment because deficiencies usually develop in the first few weeks of feeding.

Section 4 **Differential Diagnosis**

Chapter 7

Diseases That Can Mimic Eating Disorders

Study Questions

- *Should you order specific tests to rule out cancer, malabsorption, inflammatory bowel disease, celiac disease, hypoadrenalism, and hyperthyroidism in patients who are referred to you with the diagnosis of anorexia nervosa?*

The diagnosis of an eating disorder (ED) should be made by identifying the core cognitions and behaviours. It cannot be made by any laboratory test; neither can it be made solely by excluding other diagnoses. The difficulty in making the diagnosis often comes from an inadequate history owing to the limited knowledge of the health care professional or the fear and denial of the patient. If the patient denies cognitions or behaviours associated with an ED, information must be obtained in other ways.

- Collateral history (a relative or partner).
- Observation of the patient in a controlled setting.
- Comparison with the records of other health care professionals.
- Asking questions that actively challenge cognitions.
  - For example, the following questions may be put to the patient. Your question, "Picture yourself at a large buffet dinner that has sliced raw vegetables, potato salad, fruit, bread and rolls of different kinds, sliced ham and beef, sauces and gravies, pies, and cake. What would you eat?" Patient response, "Like anyone else, I would be pleased to eat at the buffet and would most certainly help myself." When pressured to give further particulars regarding what they would eat, they might say, "Some vegetables, perhaps a roll." Thus, they reveal their aversion to fatty and high-calorie foods because it is impossible for them to imagine eating fatty or high-calorie foods!
  - Question: you have lost 10 kg. If I could wave a magic wand and instantly put 10 kg of fat on your body, would that be all right? Response: "It would be alright… but it would, of course, have to be muscle, and it would have to go on slowly … to be healthy" (with a look of horror on their face).

What Physical Signs Help to Make the Diagnosis?

The physical signs that help to confirm the diagnosis of an ED are the appearance of emaciation in someone who seems to be otherwise full of energy, Russell's sign, erosion of the teeth, parotid and submandibular gland hypertrophy, hypercarotenaemia, lanugo hair, and erythema ab igne. Russell's sign can be confused with the scarring over the dorsum of the hand seen in porphyria cutanea tarda. Russell's sign is only present on the

Table 7.1 Tests that should be normal

Haematological	Clotting indices, platelet count
Biochemistry	Alkaline phosphatase, gamma glutamyl transferase, bilirubin
Immunological	ANA, RF, ENA, ESR, Schirmer test
Gastrointestinal	D-xylose test, C-14 breath test
Neurological	EEG, MRI of head
Endocrine	Prolactin, ACTH stimulation test, TRH stimulation test, antithyroid antibodies
Radiological	Skull radiograph, chest radiograph, abdominal radiograph, ultrasound examination of the abdomen

ACTH, adrenocorticotrophic hormone; ANA, antinuclear antibody; EEG, electroencephalograph; ENA, extractable nuclear antigen; ESR, erythrocyte sedimentation rate; MRI, magnetic resonance imaging; RF, rheumatoid factor; TRH, thyrotropin releasing hormone.

one hand used for purging, whereas in porphyria cutanea tarda it is seen on both hands. Bilateral parotid gland hypertrophy can accompany mumps, protein–calorie malnutrition of any cause, and alcoholism. Unilateral parotid gland hypertrophy is uncommon in EDs and may be a sign of infection or tumour of the parotid. However, if the patient lies on one side only while sleeping, the dependent side may be larger. Hypercarotenaemia is useful in distinguishing malabsorption (low serum carotene), from anorexia nervosa (AN; high serum carotene). Hypercarotenaemia is only seen in AN, hypothyroidism, and in children who ingest a lot of carotene. Children become hypercarotenemic because the liver that breaks down the carotene is not fully mature and therefore does not break down carotene as quickly as in adults. Lanugo hair is only seen in AN. However, this symptom cannot be used to make the diagnosis because the identification of lanugo hair is subjective.

There are a number of laboratory tests that are usually normal in AN and bulimia nervosa (Table 7.1). If any of these are abnormal, another disease process should be considered.

Psychiatric Diseases That Can Mimic EDs

Major depressive disorder should be considered in the differential diagnosis of AN, especially in patients older than 40 years of age. A major depressive disorder may be associated with weight loss, a loss of appetite, and a loss of motivation to eat. AN does not cause a loss of appetite. The patient with AN chooses not to eat – despite great hunger and a desire for food (although they often deny hunger). Unlike AN, major depressive disorder is not associated with an excessive concern about body shape or the caloric content of food, unless the depression is secondary to or concurrent with AN or bulimia nervosa. Unlike major depressive disorder, people with AN are pleased about their weight loss.

Obsessive–compulsive disorder and psychoses are occasionally misdiagnosed as an ED. Obsessional symptoms (e.g., fear of eating contaminated food or decreased food intake owing to the urge to chew each mouthful a specific number of times) may also account for weight loss. As always, a thorough psychiatric history is necessary before making a diagnosis.

Loss of appetite and hypophagia are seen in many physical disorders, as well as in depression and dementia, and may sometimes occur in the context of a severe personality disturbance. Hyperphagia is characteristic of certain organic disorders, including hypothalamic tumour, the Klein–Levin syndrome, and Prader–Willi syndrome.

Anxiety about eating with others may be an expression of social phobia, and repeated spontaneous vomiting may also be anxiety related. Such disturbances of eating are not EDs as such, because they are secondary either to a general medical disorder or to another psychiatric condition.

Medical Diseases That Can Mimic EDs

In general, patients with an ED look and act amazingly well compared with those who have lost as much weight from a medical disorder. In the absence of behavioural or cognitive indicators of AN, the clinician may suspect a somatic cause of weight loss such as diabetes mellitus, hyperthyroidism, Addison disease, human immunodeficiency virus/acquired immune deficiency syndrome, chronic infectious disease, carcinoma, malabsorption (e.g., sprue), Crohn's disease or a chronic debilitating disease. However, it is not advisable to encourage extensive and invasive medical investigations if the patient's symptoms can be explained adequately by the diagnosis of AN or another ED.

Addison Disease

Addison disease usually presents with weight loss over months to a few years accompanied by lethargy, slightly elevated serum potassium, and slightly low serum sodium. The stimulation test of cortisol measures the response of the serum cortisol to an injection of adrenocorticotrophic hormone. A doubling of the baseline serum cortisol or a peak serum cortisol of more than 500 I.U. indicates normal adrenal function and excludes Addison disease. Glucocorticoid use, other than dexamethasone, will interfere with test results.

Malabsorption

The gold standard test to exclude malabsorption is the standard faecal fat test. One hundred grams of fat must be ingested daily for 6 days, with stools collected on the last 3 days, for the standard faecal fat test. Adults normally absorb more than 95 per cent of the fat that they ingest. However, patients with and ED are usually unwilling to ingest 100 g of fat a day. A modified test can be performed in the same way with 50 g of fat a day. The D-xylose test, which is easy to perform, is a screening test for small bowel malabsorption. D-xylose, administered as an oral fluid, is a monosaccharide that is absorbed directly in the small bowel, enters the blood, and is then excreted in the urine. Small bowel malabsorption or rapid transit through the small bowel decreases the absorption and the resulting serum and urine tests.

Thyroid Dysfunction

The serum thyroid-stimulating hormone regulates the thyroid hormone level in the blood like a thermostat. When thyroid hormone is too high, as in hyperthyroidism or when taking too much thyroid hormone, the thyroid-stimulating hormone will be low, or "turn off". When thyroid hormone is too low, in hypothyroidism, the thyroid-stimulating hormone will be high, or "turned on".

Hyperthyroidism can cause food to move through the bowel too quickly, causing malabsorption. Patients with AN who become hyperthyroid may paradoxically experience increased appetite, weight gain, and consequently feelings of loss of control of weight and shape. Successful treatment of the hyperthyroidism reverses the increase in appetite.

Inflammatory Bowel Disease

Crohn's disease may be associated with anorexia, lethargy, and a depressed mood – sometimes with few gastrointestinal symptoms, especially in teenagers. Consultation should be made to a gastroenterologist if inflammatory bowel disease is suspected. If the patient has inflammatory bowel disease that was diagnosed previously, the treating gastroenterologist should be consulted because of the potential overlap of symptoms, complications, and medication interactions.

Celiac Disease

Celiac disease is commonly seen in association with an ED. Celiac disease (gluten-induced enteropathy, sprue) often presents with an isolated deficiency of a nutrient or weight loss that is so gradual as to go unnoticed, with little or no associated diarrhoea. Celiac is now a common disease. It results from both environmental (gluten) and genetic factors (human leukocyte antigen and non-human leukocyte antigen genes]. Importantly, patients with celiac disease often complain of intolerance and allergies to numerous foods that interfere with recovery. Many foods, medications, and even chewing gum contain gluten. Consultation from a dietitian and a pharmacist is, therefore, essential if the diagnosis is made. Immunoglobulin A tissue transglutaminase antibody is a blood test that can be used to screen for celiac disease. A small bowel biopsy is still the gold standard for diagnosis of celiac disease.

Constitutionally Low Body Fat

Constitutionally low body fat means that the patient has low body weight not owing to an ED or any other disease. These patients characteristically have always been thin, have tried to gain weight without success, and regard themselves as being less attractive because of their thinness, but have normal physiological function, including menstruation. They should have occult causes of weight loss excluded and their bone density measured because this value is low in some patients.

Cancer

Cancer can present with weight loss, vomiting, sweats, loss of appetite, change in taste, aversion to food, and other symptoms that might suggest an ED. The patient with cancer is compliant and concerned. Very rarely, a cancer will present with a marked increase in appetite, leading to bingeing and progressive weight gain.

Munchausen Syndrome

Patients with an ED can present with concomitant Munchausen syndrome or Munchausen syndrome by proxy. Munchhausen syndrome is a recurrent, simulated, feigned illness; a form of pathological lying in which patients describe very wild, overstated

Table 7.2 The clinical presentation of Munchausen syndrome

System	Presentation
Gastrointestinal	Diarrhoea (laxatives) Abdominal pain Vomiting Nausea Dehydration
Pulmonary	Pneumonia
Cardiac	Torsade de pointes
Neurological	Unwitnessed head injury and amnesia Vertigo Delirium
Endocrine	Hyperglycaemia (falsely recorded high blood glucose levels made by parent) Hypokalaemia (laxatives)
Infectious	Factitious fever of unknown origin Bacteraemia (injecting unclean water intravenously)
Dermatological	Cutting wrist, arms, and abdomen
Psychiatric	Depressive and hypomanic episodes Psychotic episode with hallucinations Hysterical conversion reaction Threatened suicide
Other	Self-injurious behaviours Pseudocyesis Ruptured her own membranes because tired of being pregnant Overdose on pills Unnecessary surgical procedures

stories (pseudologia fantastica) and seeking advice from different hospitals or in different cities. Munchhausen syndrome by proxy is defined as an illness fabricated by a parent or someone who is in loco parentis (acts as or in lieu of parental presence). The child frequently is presented for medical assessments, the perpetrator denies knowledge, and the acute signs and symptoms of the illness cease when the child is separated from the perpetrator. Munchausen syndrome and EDs share a number of signs and symptoms: self-injurious behaviour, manipulation, splitting, physical complaints, multiple admissions, noncompliance, and giving false information. The presentation of Munchausen syndrome or Munchausen syndrome by proxy in patients with EDs is presented in Table 7.2.

At the time of diagnosis, Munchausen syndrome or Munchausen syndrome by proxy has, in retrospect, usually been present for years. The essential step is to consider the diagnosis. Once considered, making the diagnosis remains difficult because the available clinical evidence is often absent, contradictory, or of uncertain importance. In Figure 8.1, we present an algorithm of the diagnostic process. In step 1, other medical or psychiatric diseases are excluded. All past medical records should be searched for clues. In step 2, admissions with no diagnosis and surgeries with no pathology are documented. In step 3,

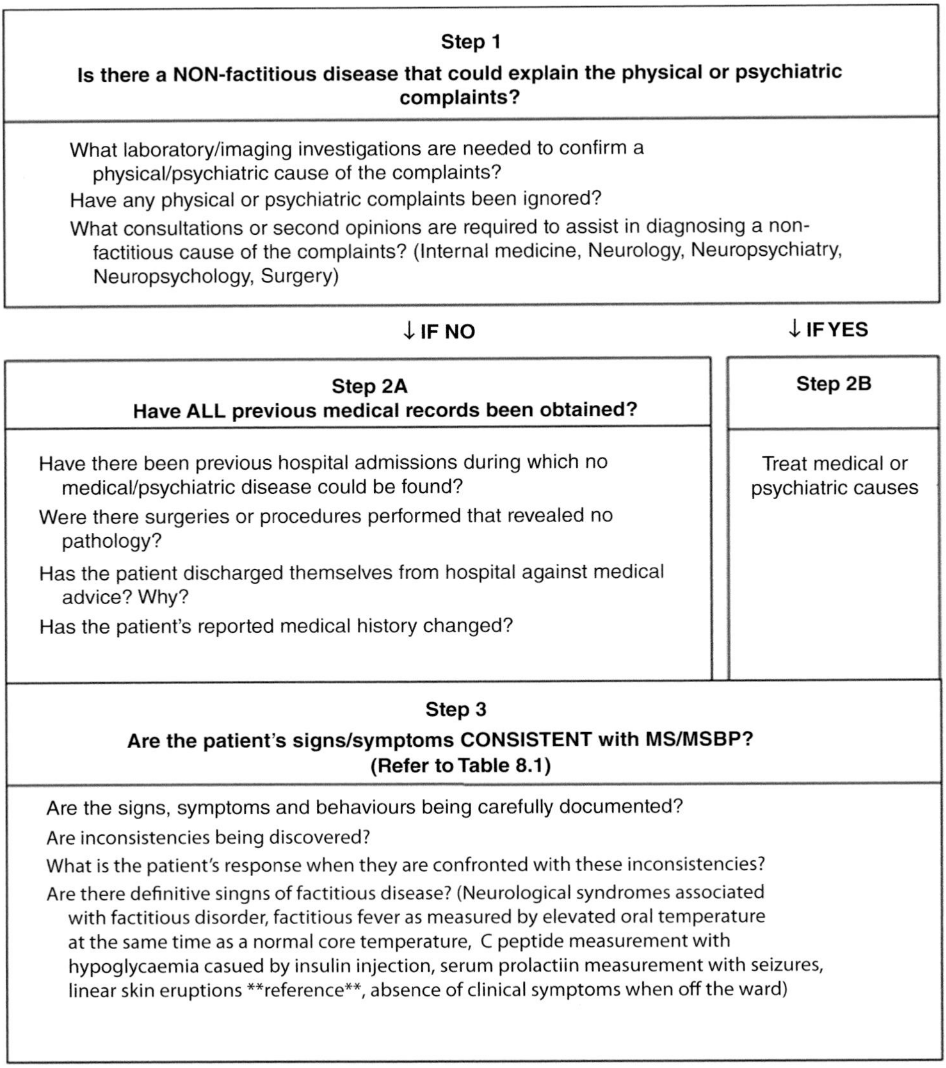

Step 1 **Is there a NON-factitious disease that could explain the physical or psychiatric complaints?**
What laboratory/imaging investigations are needed to confirm a physical/psychiatric cause of the complaints? Have any physical or psychiatric complaints been ignored? What consultations or second opinions are required to assist in diagnosing a non-factitious cause of the complaints? (Internal medicine, Neurology, Neuropsychiatry, Neuropsychology, Surgery)

↓ IF NO ↓ IF YES

Step 2A **Have ALL previous medical records been obtained?**	**Step 2B**
Have there been previous hospital admissions during which no medical/psychiatric disease could be found? Were there surgeries or procedures performed that revealed no pathology? Has the patient discharged themselves from hospital against medical advice? Why? Has the patient's reported medical history changed?	Treat medical or psychiatric causes

Step 3 **Are the patient's signs/symptoms CONSISTENT with MS/MSBP?** **(Refer to Table 8.1)**
Are the signs, symptoms and behaviours being carefully documented? Are inconsistencies being discovered? What is the patient's response when they are confronted with these inconsistencies? Are there definitive singns of factitious disease? (Neurological syndromes associated with factitious disorder, factitious fever as measured by elevated oral temperature at the same time as a normal core temperature, C peptide measurement with hypoglycaemia casued by insulin injection, serum prolactiin measurement with seizures, linear skin eruptions **reference**, absence of clinical symptoms when off the ward)

Figure 7.1 Munchausen syndrome algorithm for diagnosis.

signs, symptoms, and behaviours that are consistent with a factitious disorder are document. Munchausen syndrome or Munchausen syndrome by proxy in patients with EDs is presented in Figure 7.1.

Implications for Health Care Professionals

- The diagnosis of an ED is usually made by history and may be confirmed by physical signs like parotid hypertrophy, lanugo hair, hypercarotenaemia, and Russell's sign.
- Patients may present or be sent for diagnoses who have another disorder – although this is unusual. They may also have an ED and another disorder. Most commonly,

one disorder began first, like depression or trauma, which precipitated the weight loss that led to the ED.

- Consider an alternate or second diagnosis when another disorder began first, with worsening of the ED for no apparent reason, or if the signs or symptoms of the ED changed. For example, if celiac disease complicates an ED, there may be worsening of malnutrition, a change in foods that are avoided, or new deficiencies.
- Munchausen syndrome is very rare. If it is suspected, the first step is to verify the past history of disease.

Patient Information

- Some patients with an ED will have their disease precipitated by or worsened by another psychiatric or medical disease. If this is the case, finding the other disorder and treating it may hasten recovery.

Chapter 8

Course and Prognosis

The outcome of eating disorders (EDs) is related to the strength of the maintaining factors and whether they have flourished untreated over time. Secondary effects can lead to a permanent imprint on the individual either because normal development is derailed, for example, leading to immaturity in the social brain and other secondary disabilities that may impair recovery; or neuroplastic changes within the brain can produce a dysregulation of appetite, for example, reward sensitisation.

Anorexia Nervosa

The outcome of treatment of adolescents is good with approximately 80 per cent achieving a good recovery. However, the outcome for those who have had the illness longer than 3 years is less good and less than 50 per cent of these have a good outcome. More than 30 per cent develop binge eating in some form. Social and physical disability remains problematic, with 20 per cent reliant on state benefits. A 1995 meta-analysis found an aggregate mortality rate of 5.6 per cent per decade for anorexia nervosa (AN), substantially greater than that reported for female psychiatric patients and the general population. Approximately one-half of the deaths result from medical complications and the rest result from suicide. Treatment in specialised centres probably improves the outcome; the mortality rate in areas/cohorts without access to specialised service is higher.

Poor prognostic factors for AN include a long duration of symptoms, especially with no treatment; developmental problems including childhood eating; compulsive and family difficulties; vomiting; bulimia; obsessive–compulsive disorder; sexual problems; a low body mass index; high intensity of eating psychopathology; and difficulty gaining weight despite treatment.

Poor Prognostic Factors for AN

- Later onset.
- Long duration of illness.
- Low minimum weight.
- Binge/purge behaviour.
- Personality difficulties.
- Poor family relationships.

Good Prognostic Factors for AN

- Early onset.
- Short duration of illness.
- Good family relationships.

Bulimia Nervosa

More than 50 per cent of patients with bulimia have a good reduction of symptoms with evidence-based treatment. Approximately 10 per cent to 20 per cent continue to meet clinical criteria for up to 10 years. It is common for 'recovered' patients to continue experiencing the core cognitive distortions that define the disorder and to suffer from persistent social disability, with an increased risk of addiction and major depression.

The prognostic features for bulimia nervosa include duration of symptoms, high levels of shape and weight concern, low self-esteem, impulsivity, personality difficulty, and poor social adjustment. Substance use comorbidity has a detrimental effect on all forms of ED.

Poor Prognostic Factors for Bulimia Nervosa

- Psychiatric comorbidity.
- Severity of symptoms.
- Impulsive personality traits.
- Substance misuse.

Implications for Health Care Professionals

- AN was recognised as a medical condition from the nineteenth century.
- The bulimic forms of EDs emerged in the last half of the twentieth century.
- People with AN are at high risk of developing bingeing and purging with irresistible, insatiable urges to eat.
- Diagnostic classification based on current symptoms alone may be less helpful than a formulation developed from a consideration of traits, symptoms, and life story.
- Patients with EDs and their carers are often frustrated, ashamed, and guilty because there is a widespread misperception that their illness is either self-imposed or caused by the family. Medical professionals need to debunk this myth.
- An important part of the process of engagement with an individual is to develop a broad ranging individualised formulation.

Patient Information

- EDs are complex developmental problems caused by a mixture of innate and acquired risk factors.
- Many of the factors that increase the risk of developing EDs are no one's fault. They include genetic risks and events that occur early in development, which set the stress system to be more sensitive and the metabolic system to be unstable.
- The thinking styles that increase the risk of an ED are helpful in many aspects of life. For example, they facilitate tasks that require diligence, detailed analysis, and

focused application. However, they become harmful when they become largely focused on dietary restriction or aesthetic judgments about the body.

- People with EDs can easily lose sight of the big picture that they need to create a fulfilling and enriching life. They may require help from concerned others to develop this perspective.
- The consequences of an ED can affect many parts of life. Without effective help, it is easy to become trapped by the ED.
- Starvation, stress, vomiting, and intermittent sugar rushes can produce addictive changes in the brain.

Section 5 Course and Prognosis

Chapter 9

Agreeing on a Goal Weight

Study Question

- *How will your team determine the goal weight and who among the team will monitor the goal weight and give the patient information any change in it?*

The goal weight must ultimately be that which restores the patient's physical and mental health. It is preferable to use total body fat as the measure of weight restoration, because measurements of total body fat are less changed by lean body mass, fluid, faeces, water loading, surreptitious use of weights, body habitus, and foetus – if the patient is pregnant. The physiological measure of restoration of body fat is menses or dominant follicles in women. There is no similar measure in men, but there is usually recovery of libido and an increase in muscle strength.

Measuring total body fat with anthropometrics with skin fold callipers with parallel weight measurements in best. This step allows the patient to follow the measurement they will use later, weight. It also shows them that the marked variations in body weight are not due to body fat – because it changes slowly and without the marked variations of weight. For women from 16–29 years of age, I use 22 per cent total body fat as the goal. Above 30 years of age, I use 26 per cent with the Durnin and Womersley chart. For males between 16 and 20 years of age, I use 14 per cent. However, if anorexic rumination and cognitive and physical abnormalities persist, the "normal" weight has not been reached.

Setting the patient's "normal, projected, goal, or restored" weight can become the focus of discussion early in treatment. This discussion can remove focus from recovery, split the team, and cause the patient to lose confidence in their treatment team. This situation can be avoided by sticking to a standard plan for all patients that is logical, easily understood, and supported by all staff. The standard plan will be different between treatment teams. It may vary depending on the measurements available, the setting (inpatient, residential, outpatient, availability of professionals from different health care backgrounds), and the philosophy of the program. But, within that treatment team it is best to stick the same standard plan.

The following guidelines are suggested to answer the question, "What is my goal weight?", both for within the team and with the patient. Ask the patient whether they agree to the following statements and goals.

1. The eating disorder (ED) has taken control of their life. The goal of treatment is to give you back that control.
2. Our goal is for your weight to normalise gradually. You will be told your weight (or your body mass index [BMI] or your per cent body fat). You will be given the results only at the time we take the measures routinely.

3. If you decide you do not want to know – we will respect that and not tell you. However, we will still take and record the measurements.
4. If you change your mind and want to know your results, you must wait until the next time that measurements are taken to be told. We want to make sure you are certain about your decision.
5. Our goal for you is health of mind and body. This means that your bones, brain, menses (for women), and all other bodily processes should function normally. It also means that you will have recovered your ability to think, remember, have self-esteem, and achieve your educational or work goals.
6. Your weight is made up of fluid, muscle, faeces, and urine, as well as fatty tissue. Sixty per cent of your body weight is water. Any weight fluctuations that occur during refeeding are like those that you may have experienced before menstrual periods, owing to fluid retention.
7. Usually, the return of regular menses, if they have stopped, means that you have reached a healthy weight. However, the occasional single period may occur during weight recovery with severe stress, thyroid dysfunction, or rapidly changing hormones.
8. If your periods do not start when we estimate you are at a healthy weight, we can order a pelvic ultrasound examination to look for dominant follicles. Dominant follicles, which have a diameter of 2 cm of greater, are diagnostic of normal hormonal cycling and therefore a healthy weight.
9. You will never want to be obese. Even if you fully "weight recover", you will continue to have a life-long overconcern about weight and shape. Your concern about weight and shape will continue to be greater than those without EDs.
10. Our estimate for the weight (BMI or per cent body fat) that will optimise your health is. . ..

Implications for Health Care Professionals

1. Decide on your team's standard use of measuring weight gain and stick to it. Also decide who will take the measurements, whether there will be a constant time or day and dress code for the patient, and who can change the protocol.
2. Although it is vogue to use BMI, do not use it. It was developed as an epidemiological tool to allow weight to be displayed standardised to height. For each individual whose height is not going to change during the measurement period, it decreases the ability of the patient and team to understand the many causes of fluctuations in weight like oedema, ingestion of water, and hiding weights under clothes. BMI is not magic but, like magic, it distracts the attention of the patient and health care professional.
3. Focus the patient on recovery of health, brain function, self-esteem, and control.

Patient Information

1. The ED has taken control of their life. The goal of treatment is to give you back that control. Our plan is to help you gain weight gradually and you will be given the results, unless you decide you do not want to know them.

2. Your goal is health – health of mind and body. This means that your bones, brain, menses (for women), and all other bodily processes should function normally.
   It also means that you will have recovered your ability to think, remember, possess good self-esteem, and achieve your educational or work goals.
3. Your tissues, like body fat and muscle, will normalise gradually during treatment. Your weight is made up of fluid, muscle, faeces, and urine, as well as fatty tissue. Sixty per cent of your body weight is water. Any weight fluctuations that occur during refeeding are like those that you may have experienced before menstrual periods, owing to fluid retention.
4. You will never want to be obese. Even if you fully "weight recover" you will continue to have a life-long overconcern about weight and shape. Your concern about weight and shape will continue to be greater than those without EDs.

Section 5 Course and Prognosis

Chapter 10

Reducing the Risk of Death

Case

- *A 35-year-old woman with anorexia nervosa reads that her life expectancy may be shortened by 22 years if she does not recover from the disease.*

The standardised mortality ratio (SMR) compares the death rate of those with a disease with the death rate in the general population, corrected (stratified) by sex and age. An SMR of 1 means the death rate of that disease is no different than the general population. The SMR for schizophrenia is 2.7. The SMR is 10.5 for anorexia nervosa (AN) and 2.0 for bulimia nervosa. AN has the highest SMR of any psychiatric disorder.

One-half of the deaths from AN are due to suicide and one-half result from a medical cause. Most medical deaths are related to starvation, which can cause failure of every body system. Heart rhythm problems, bacterial infections, hypoglycaemia, cachexia, gastric disease, liver failure, bone marrow failure, pulmonary emboli, myocardial infarction, and central pontine myelolysis have all been reported as causes of death in AN.

Life Expectancy

The life expectancy of patients who are diagnosed with AN is decreased by 22 years on average. This rate is similar to many forms of cancer. This statistic may motivate the patient to recover.

How to Decrease the Risk of Death

The major challenge in the medical management of patients with eating disorders (EDs) is to better predict arrhythmias that can cause death. A rapid normalisation of heart rate variability is likely the most important factor – in combination with other factors like prolonged QTc interval, low serum potassium, magnesium, or phosphorus.

The 'fight-or-flight' nervous system in the brain – the autonomic nervous system – regulates organs that are not under conscious control. Thus, the heart, lungs, bowel, bladder, and blood vessels, among others, are regulated by the autonomic nervous system. When there is a very stressful situation, the autonomic nervous system will speed up the heart rate, concentrating blood flow to the heart and brain and away from the extremities, and cause contraction of the bladder and bowel followed by a pause in their function. In patients with an ED, there is often a wide variability of heart rate over time. This in itself does not increase the risk of sudden death. However, low heart rate variability caused by a rapid change in autonomic function does predispose to arrhythmia. Table 10.1 lists ways of decreasing the risk of death in EDs.

Table 10.1 How to decrease the risk of death

Cause of Death	When It Occurs	How to Treat or Reduce Risk
Hypoglycaemia	Increase in caloric intake	Eat small meals every 4 hours Avoid simple sugars Home testing of blood sugar 'Test' with orange juice
Cardiac arrhythmia	Low potassium, magnesium, phosphorus Change in heart rate variability	Monitor during refeeding Routine supplementation Increase supplementation if levels are decreasing With intermittent perspiration, inappropriate increase or decrease heart rate, bowel and bladder function Decrease exercise, slow refeeding, consider a centrally acting beta-blocker
Infection	Low weight	Treat all bacterial and fungal infections that occur at low weight as you would in the immunosuppressed Investigate possible infections more thoroughly and treat more aggressively
Suicide	Loss of hope Improved cognition Rapid weight gain Loss of trust	Reestablish rapport Explain that feelings of hopelessness commonly increase when the 'fog clears' Explain that they can lose the weight again if they want Recovery is not an amputation

The Law, Ethics, and Clinical Decision Analysis

Because a core feature of AN is the fixed idea that gain weight is terrifying, these patients are often highly ambivalent about the need for treatment. Mental health legislation is used to provide compulsory treatment if the risk is high.

Increasingly, lawyers, ethicists, epidemiologists, and even the politicians help medical practitioners to decide whether a patient should be forced to undergo treatment. It is paramount that the practitioner be able to present the risks and benefits of the alternatives to the patient and these experts. Clinical decision analysis forces us to make the various treatment decisions more understandable.

How to Use Clinical Decision Analysis

Ethic clinical decision analysis is the graphical representation of the probabilities of possible outcomes (Bayes' theorem). It can be used to help make treatment decisions, like whether to involuntarily feed or admit to the hospital a patient with AN. A decision tree is constructed with each treatment option assigned to one arm. The decision is made by comparing the values calculated for each arm by simple arithmetic or the decision analysis computer program.

The analysis requires all the options to have separate arms representing them and each arm having a numerical value and a numerical probability. The numerical value is assigned to each option based on the known value or relative benefit of the possible outcomes. For example, death is usually scored as 0 and good health is scored as 1. The numerical probability of each outcome is estimated from the literature or experience. It may be a range, for example, 0.2–0.6 per cent or 20–60 per cent.

What if there is uncertainty about the probabilities and relative benefits that are being used? Would a different number change the decision? If the clinical team disagrees about the estimate of a probability or relative benefit, you can calculate each of the possible outcomes separately or perform a sensitivity analysis. A sensitivity analysis produces a range of outcomes over a range of probabilities or values; from those, the most favourable to the least favourable can be determined.

Implications for Health Care Professionals

1. Focus on decreasing the risk of death.
2. When confronted by lawyers, ethicists, and politicians who have come to tell you not to treat a patient, use a clinical decision analysis, or at least a design tree, to present the options with their probabilities of outcomes.
3. Although the risk of various causes of death continues to be debated, decrease all risks of death that you can.

Patient Information

1. The life expectancy of patients who are diagnosed with AN is decreased by 22 years on average.
2. See Table 10.1 to discover ways to decrease your risk of death.

Chapter 11

Evidence-Based Approach for the Treatment of Eating Disorders

Introduction

In this chapter, we synthesise and review the evidence base relating to treatment. However, the literature is not evenly spread across the disorders. The evidence base for the treatment of anorexia nervosa (AN) is meagre in contrast with that available for the binge eating forms of eating disorders (EDs). Cognitive–behavioural therapy has been found to be effective in the management of the binge EDs in about 50 per cent of cases. However the management of AN is more complex because the type of case involved is broad, ranging from child to adult, dependent to independent, high to low medical risk, and early onset to persistent. There is, therefore, less evidence that can be applied to an individual case. Managing AN requires both clinical judgment and skilled negotiation. The latter is necessary because people with AN are highly resistant to change.

Psychological, pharmacological, and some physical (e.g., massage) treatments have been examined, as have different forms of service (inpatient, outpatient, specialist, nonspecialist, etc.). This area is rapidly changing and cannot be captured in a text book; it is important to refer to guidelines or recent systematic reviews.

In the second part of the chapter, we describe the art of developing a plan of care, which is particularly relevant to AN, but is also needed for complex forms of binge eating associated with diabetes, addictions, and pregnancy.

Summarising the Evidence

This is a rapidly changing area; therefore, it may be necessary to refer to guidelines and updated systematic reviews. Some of the national guidelines synthesise the evidence in a systematic way, for example, the UK National Institute for Health and Care Excellence guidelines. Other countries publish their own guidelines based on different processes for generating the evidence; for example, guidelines in the United States provide a narrative review. The overall conclusions that can be synthesised from the evidence are shown in Table 11.1.

Involving the family in treatment produces a greater level of change in adolescent AN, but the form (multifamily groups, individual families, or parents separate from patient) or even the amount by which the family/parents are involved is uncertain. (For example, seeing the family/parents separately from the individual produces greater change in families who are highly stressed by their role.) Specialist forms of treatment for adults with AN seem to produce more change than treatment delivered by generic therapists. However, there is no evidence yet that the form and content of the treatments has an impact on outcome. Medication does not appear to have an impact on change in AN.

Table 11.1 Summary of the evidence for treatments of EDs

ED	Treatment Summary	Comment
AN	Service form (inpatient vs. outpatient)	Short inpatient stays for adolescents followed by day care or FBT is as effective as protracted in patient stay.
	Family (multigroups, individual) carer skills training, or separated	Multigroups and separated (parents and child seen apart) produce similar outcomes to traditional family therapy and may be superior for cases with high expressed emotion. Early intervention for adolescent AN improves outcome. Carer skill training improves carer well-being and can improve patient outcomes.
	Individual (CBT, MANTRA, IPT, focal)	All produce similar low–moderate levels of change. Treatment with a nonspecialist dietitian or psychiatrist is less effective.
	Medication (antidepressants, antipsychotics) in acute phase or to prevent relapse	No/small effects.
Bulimia nervosa	Family	Moderate effects in adolescents – less rapid change than guided CBT.
	Individual (CBT, IPT, DBT)	CBT produces large and rapid effects which are sustained.
	Medication (antidepressants, mood stabilisers)	Moderate to large effects in the short term.
Binge eating disorder	Individual (CBT, IPT, DBT)	Moderate to large change in binges.
	Behavioural weight loss treatments	Moderate to large effects on binges and weight.
	Medication (antidepressants, mood stabilisers, antiobesity agents, lisdexamphetamine)	Moderate to large effects on bingeing and weight.

Abbreviations: AN, anorexia nervosa; CBT, cognitive-behavioural therapy (the focus of treatment is changing thinking and meaning with aim of changing emotions and behaviour); DBT, dialectical–behavioural therapy (treatment focused on finding a balance between acceptance and change, especially relating to emotions); ED, eating disorder; Focal, focused therapy (this form of treatment focuses on interpersonal relationships and the therapeutic alliance); IPT, interpersonal therapy (this therapy formulates problems in terms of a variety of interpersonal challenges or difficulties); MANTRA, Maudsley Outpatient Treatment for Anorexia Nervosa (the focus is on interpersonal relationships and how patterns of thoughts, feelings and interactions can become fixed in an unhelpful manner and managing extreme personality traits such as obsessive compulsive or autistic spectrum traits).
Nonadherence or protocol violations: Failure to engage in treatment or dropping out of treatment is common in all treatments but especially those involving medication or inpatient care. Some cases fail to respond to treatment and their health and safety are at risk and so they may be rescued to a higher intensity of treatment.

Cognitive–behavioural therapy and pharmacotherapy can produce large changes in binge eating behaviours. Nevertheless, approximately 50 per cent of patients fail to respond to these treatments. However, it is possible to detect such nonresponders early in the course of treatment, because they fail to respond within the first few weeks of treatment. Therefore, there is interest in treatments that offer a different focus.

Pathways of Care

Describing the pathway through care in AN is complex, because there is such a broad variability in the clinical presentation (child vs. adult, dependent/independent, high vs. low risk, resistant/motivated, etc.). There is more uniformity in the presentation of the binge forms of EDs, and most are managed with outpatient care.

However, patients with other addictions, diabetes, and pregnancy may have further problems that might need different styles of management. If other addictions are present, it is helpful to work with them all in synchrony. An abstinence-based model may be appropriate for the other addictions, but cannot fit for food; however, a useful strategy is to avoid highly palatable foods containing high levels of fat and sugar and replace them with a diet in which blood sugar levels are stable throughout the day.

People with diabetes commonly use so-called insulin purging; this act is when they cut back on their insulin. Sugar is not taken up for metabolism, but is lost in the urine. In the short term, this strategy can cause metabolic and fluid balance chaos and in the long term accelerates the development of diabetic complications. Thus, the management of the diabetes needs to be a focus alongside that of the ED.

Pregnancy is fraught with anxiety in people with EDs and causes symptoms of EDs to re-emerge. One consequence can be for them to 'let themselves go', and pull off all dietary restraint during the pregnancy and then go on a stringent diet after birth. Not only does this plan foster the maintenance of the ED, but it may through the mechanism of foetal programming produce metabolic consequences for the offspring. The aim should be to stabilise sugar levels and eating patterns as much as possible.

Early Intervention

In the ideal scenario, EDs are recognised and treated in their early stages; however, the major obstacles preventing this happening is that individuals with AN characteristically do not acknowledge their difficulties, and people with bulimia nervosa or BED may be embarrassed to describe their symptoms. New forms of service delivery (e.g., web based), as well as forms of self-help with or without guidance may overcome treatment barriers for bulimia nervosa, whereas working through the family can be used for adolescent AN.

AN: General

The Form of Service for AN

In many countries, clinical practice with AN has changed over the past several decades from extended inpatient hospitalisations to a greater emphasis on outpatient treatment. Therefore, in contemporary practice, a stepped care approach to treatment is generally recommended, with inpatient care reserved for those at high risk and poor psychosocial resources. This treatment is more acceptable to patients and has economic advantages.

A counterargument from those who advocate more intensive care is that the outcome with AN is improved if weight is restored to the normal range and this goal can be more reliably attained with inpatient care. Current guidelines in the United States suggest that intensive 24-hour care should be used when the body mass index (BMI) drops below 16 or when weight decreases by 20 per cent, whereas in the UK a lower (undefined) threshold is used and outpatient treatment is recommended as the first step. In our National Health Service practice in London, we find that about 50 per cent of those who have a body mass index of less than 15 will require admission because they are unable to make progress as an outpatient.

The Form of Treatment for AN

Practice recommendations from professional organisations emphasise the importance of a multidisciplinary approach including medical, nutrition, and psychological components. For the type of psychological treatments that are of value, see Chapter 13.

Planning Treatment for People with EDs

The first stage of planning treatment for people with EDs involves a detailed psychological and physical assessment of the individual and the family. This assessment is followed by feedback, during which a joint formulation is developed. The range of risk, maturation, and motivation is wide. The risks and resources, and hence prognosis, for each case need to be evaluated carefully. Treatment needs to be tailored for the individual and her or his family with regular adjustments made over time, depending on progress. An outline of how this balance can be made is shown in Table 11.2.

The only simple and fixed aspect of treatment planning is the need to continuously monitor progress by measuring medical risk and weight (for AN). In the case of AN, it is important that strategies to prevent the evolution of bulimia nervosa be in place.

Matching the intensity and type of treatment to need involves a careful risk assessment of medical, clinical, and psychosocial factors. There is a need to balance the severity

Table 11.2 Setting the agenda of treatments, balancing risks and resources

Risk	Readiness	Resource	Procedure
High	Discuss legal rules and medical feedback relating to importance of change for health and safety reasons Elicit where change can occur, e.g., inpatient vs. outpatient. Elicit who can help: family/friends vs. nurses.	Prepare, plan, and liaison for intensive care. Inform network, carers, medical team (legal context).	Monitor frequently. Visit the unit. Meet with carers. Outline legal framework and conditions.
Low	Ensure nutrition and eating is on the agenda; however, there can be some choice of target behaviours and goal setting.	Discuss what would happen if high risk developed. Offer the option of working with the family.	Monitor regularly. Develop the formulation.

of the weight loss against the resources that the patient has to implement renutrition and to judge whether starvation requires acute management. The plan of management may include day and outpatient care with complex mixes of types of therapy and number of hours over a variety of durations and with an individual and various members of her or his family.

Confidentiality

Issues of confidentiality need to be considered. AN in particular is highly visible in the social arena and cannot be considered as a totally confidential matter between doctor and patient. Also, starvation impacts on capacity and decision making and has legal implications if there is high risk and responsible others become involved in such a scenario. The details of therapy can be privileged and confidential; however, the broad aspects information about EDs in general can and should be shared with carers. It is good practice to discuss how risk will be managed. If the risk is high this plan of management needs to be shared with carers.

Intensive Forms of Treatment: Inpatient and Day Patient

Inpatient care is needed if there is high risk, low motivation, and low resources (see Table 11.1). There are cultural differences according to national services and across units as to when inpatient care is used and how much this is conducted under the control of the mental health act. Inpatient treatment in a unit with skilled staff can successfully produce weight gain and improve safety. However, the imposed behaviour change may not be associated with changes in the core psychopathology and weight loss and relapse into active AN after discharge is common. Also, there is often poor adherence to inpatient care and early discharge. There is a risk of institutionalisation, especially for young patients and admission in this group should be as short as possible. This opens up the question of what should be the goals of inpatient care. If the goal is to restore weight into the normal range, then admissions either have to be protracted (too high a rate of weight gain, e.g., more than 2 kg/week may be both physically and psychologically aversive). On the other hand, if the goal of the admission is to safeguard risk or to give the family respite, or support the initial steps of behaviour change then shorter admissions can be used. People with severe enduring AN (i.e., long duration and with extreme weight loss) may benefit from longer treatment that initially involves hospital care integrated with rehabilitation. There is a lack of evidence to support this clinical decision making and most countries follow their own guidelines.

The following clinical case gives an example of how the negotiation of risk and its management can be addressed early on in treatment. The therapist is using the principles of motivational interviewing and is sharing the medical work up of risk as a form of feedback.

Clinical Case

Susan is a 25-year-old nurse who developed AN at the age of 12. (Her mother had also had AN in her youth). She had had phases in her life when she had made a partial recovery, for example, when she went to a mixed sixth form college to do her A levels. She was much less pressured then and she made some good friends in this period.

However, when she went to university she became somewhat isolated and more focused on her work, and lost weight again in the first 2 years. Her tutor insisted that she undergo treatment and she had an episode of inpatient care. She was able to return to her course after having made a great deal of progress. She chose to specialise in paediatric nursing and had been working on the neonatal intensive care unit. However, she found this job very stressful. The medical team that she worked with was unsupportive and highly critical. She developed obsessive-compulsive symptoms of checking and cleaning, and her ED once again came to the fore. Her line manager suggested that she go to occupational health and from there she was referred for treatment to a specialised unit. The occupational health doctor said that she could stay at work if she was being monitored and in treatment.

When she saw the specialist ED clinician, she was somewhat guarded and not very communicative. Her BMI was 13.5 kg/m^2, but had been relatively stable over the last 6 months since other people had expressed their concern and the treatment process had been instigated. She had no myopathy (she did the squat test easily). Her blood pressure was 100/60 both lying and standing. She was anaemic with a haemoglobin of 10.5 and her white cell count was low at 3.3 cells/µl.

In this session, the ED specialist (EDS) reviews her medical status with her using the BMI chart and the medical risk form as a means of delivering feedback and social norms.

ED SPECIALIST: If we plot your BMI on this chart, you can see what zone you are in. Do you want to read what it says? (This allows S to compare herself with the normal and ED population. The chart transmits information in a neutral way. This allows the therapist to step back from a powerful role directly giving information and talking about danger and risk and to have a collaborative stance, whereby they can share the same perspective noting the objective evidence.)

SUSAN: 'Severe AN core organs show overt signs of loss of function, e.g., circulation, bone marrow, muscles.'

ED SPECIALIST: Does that fit with what you experience?

SUSAN: Not really. I feel perfectly OK. I do not know why everyone is making such a fuss.

ED SPECIALIST: Part of you is surprised that people are concerned about you because you feel OK, but another part respects their opinion and, therefore, come for treatment.

The therapist acknowledges Susan's ambivalence about treatment finishing with an affirmative comment about change.

SUSAN: My work is important for me.

ED SPECIALIST: Because of your commitment to your career, you are willing to take on board things that do not totally fit with what you experience.

Again, the therapist gives an affirmative reflection, which opens the possibility that the individual may need to take a broader perspective.

ED SPECIALIST: Let's look at this medical risk chart, if we plot your blood pressure, blood tests here you can see that we have several ticks in the high risk box. That perhaps underlines what concerns other people.

Again, by using a written feedback chart that contains normative data, the therapist can step back and yet be clear about non-negotiable areas of risk. In motivational interviewing, the position taken is that patient has full autonomy around all decisions. AN differs from alcohol disorder in that it is regarded as a mental illness that impacts the individual's health and safety and, therefore, in many countries treatment can be enforced through legislation. Some would argue that the individual's capacity to make valid decisions is impaired because of the emotional and cognitive aspects of the illness.

SUSAN: I understand what you are saying, but it does not feel like that to me.

ED SPECIALIST: The discrepancy between what you know and feel is confusing for you. It is as if the EDs play tricks with you. However, we need to work together in the context of this objective data. Does that make sense to you?

SUSAN: I suppose so.

ED SPECIALIST: In conditions of high risk, which is where you are at the moment according to this chart, the guidelines state that it is good practice to prepare for the worst and to ensure that we have your safety as a priority. That means preparing for more intensive care.

SUSAN: I don't want to go into hospital.

ED SPECIALIST: You would prefer to give outpatient treatment your best shot.

The therapist gives a positively framed reflection.

ED SPECIALIST: Let's think about what might help you to do this. How might friends and family help you stay out of hospital and turn this around?

The therapist sidesteps the resistance to talk about the hospital and gives a positively framed reflection about outpatient care. The therapist then elicits talk about change (who can help) from the patient.

SUSAN: I would prefer my parents not to be involved at the moment; it is a long way to come and it would worry them.

ED SPECIALIST: You prioritise the well-being of others above that of your own health.

Again, the therapist sidesteps entering into an argument about involving the parents and instead gives a complex reflection describing the values that drive this statement. This positive reflection is full of empathy and bolsters the individual's sense of esteem and strengthens the therapeutic alliance

ED SPECIALIST: We find that parents are desperate for information and advice and feel much better if they can help in some way. However, we can have a short experimental period in which your theory that you can turn this around yourself is put to the test. Let's examine what you are able to do in the next few days does that sound ok?

SUSAN: I think I should be able to do it.

ED SPECIALIST: It's great that you have that confidence as that will give you energy. You will need it – the battle is tough.

SUSAN: I can do it.

ED SPECIALIST: OK. Let's talk through the plan you have about making this experiment turn out the way you want. What do you think you could do about adding in more nutrition?

SUSAN: Well, I guess I could add in a cereal bar.

ED SPECIALIST: That sounds a good step. Can you tell me more about that – like when, where, and how you might be able to introduce that.

The therapist elicits how change will occur and goes into the detail of how change will be implemented. This part of the session is slow and painstaking. It is important that the patient herself does the talking, even if she is hesitant and uncertain. There needs to be time and effort for the individual to visualise the change process.

SUSAN: [Says nothing].

ED SPECIALIST: What might be the barriers that would stop you putting this into place?

SUSAN: [Says nothing].

ED SPECIALIST: Meanwhile, here is some information about the inpatient unit. We recommend that people phone and arrange to get a visit. Sometimes, it can be helpful in that it helps to be able to visualise what will need to happen if the AN proves very resistant to change. Also, some people are able to recreate some of the inpatient conditions at home and that can be helpful. When do you think you might be able to make that call and get some more information about it?

The therapist makes the consequences of failing to make the change transparent.

SUSAN: [Says nothing].

ED SPECIALIST: I will let the ward know you will ring to arrange a visit and I will ensure that your name is on the waiting list.

One week later, Susan's weight has continued to fall and blood tests show more abnormalities.

ED SPECIALIST: How did things go last week? What do you anticipate the results of the experiment have been in terms of your weight?

By asking about expected changes and measuring the reality, the therapist is able to have a measure about how much insight is present. Sometimes people anticipate that their weight will have increased by a huge amount. This will give the therapist the opportunity to challenge their perceptions about weight gain against the reality.

SUSAN: I'm not sure. I had a stomach bug. I could not eat anything on Wednesday.

ED SPECIALIST: Let's look at your weight and your physical risk markers.

SUSAN: [Says nothing].

ED SPECIALIST: It looks like it has been very tough for you to turn this around on your own.

The therapist's reflection is empathetic and by emphasising – on your own – opens the door to involving more help.

ED SPECIALIST: If we look at all this on the charts, it shows that your risk is increasing.

SUSAN: I did manage to do it some of the time – I was ill.

ED SPECIALIST: The problem is that this degree of risk gives you no leeway, and we keeping you safe have to take into account bugs, etc. Were you able to think about what I said about your family and friends and giving you help?

SUSAN: If it stops me having to go into hospital, I would do anything.

ED SPECIALIST: Can we arrange a time to meet again that might be suitable for them. Meanwhile, can you think about in what way they may be able to help.

In this case, the therapist has some time to do preparatory work before the admission, because the risk is not in the critical level. In some cases, unfortunately, there is less opportunity to set small behavioural experiments into place. It is good practice to let family members know about the legal issues and to make firm plans about an admission. All therapists working with people with EDs need to know about the procedures involved in obtaining a compulsory treatment.

Implication for Nurses

- It essential to match the treatment for AN to the needs of the individual. This process requires a careful assessment of risk and resources
- A risk assessment for AN includes consideration of several dimensions: physical health, clinical features, capacity, motivation, and social factors.
- The outcome of AN, in terms of recovery and mortality rates, is improved if the illness is short in duration; i.e., early interventions are to be recommended. However, because the onset is in early adolescence, in most cases those presenting to adult services have had the illness for more than 3 years and so the prognosis is less good.
- Severe weight loss is dangerous in the short term and leads to an adverse long-term outcome.
- Specialised treatments are more acceptable, efficacious, and cost effective in AN than nonspecialised treatment.

Chapter 12

Specific Psychological Therapies

A variety of theoretical explanatory models have been used to shape services and treatments for eating disorders (EDs). Although the nomenclature used and the emphasis given to various facets of the illness differs, many of the components used to change behaviour are similar across the models.

Therefore, rather than describing the specifics of each theoretical approach here, we describe empirically derived risk factors and discuss general change processes that are more tailored to the specific factors that predispose, precipitate, and/or perpetuate the ED. This builds on the evidence outlined in Chapter 2.

EDs are not just a simple matter of problematic eating. Rather, they involve a complex mix of emotional, cognitive, perceptual, memory, and personality factors that increase vulnerability and/or keep the behaviours stuck. These maintaining factors are a useful target because they are, by definition, currently in action, and are more accessible and available for change. The formulation derived from the assessment serves as a template for deciding which, where, how, and when behaviours should be changed.

An important part of most treatments is the development of a shared explanatory model between the therapist and the patient that describes the meaning of the illness and can help to explain the targets of change. A joint understanding of the illness may help to foster a strong therapeutic alliance.

The initial part of this chapter builds on the aetiological evidence base that was described in Chapter 2. We also discuss the interpersonal aspects of EDs, which include developing a good therapeutic alliance and working with the wider interpersonal network. The latter part of the chapter discusses the form in which treatment is delivered.

Setting the Scene for Treatment

A variety of causal explanations for EDs, with different theoretical underpinnings, are available. Thus, family, feminist, cognitive–behavioural, psychodynamic, and pharmacological approaches have all been used. However, all treatments, no matter what their orientation, need to encompass and explain the predisposing, precipitating and maintaining factors discussed in Chapter 2 (see Figure 2.1) and some components of treatment should act to buffer or remediate the impact of these factors. Thus, in addition to a focus on eating, additional facets of treatment may aim to directly moderate the harmful effects of extreme dispositions and maladaptive, coping, or emotional regulation strategies, and other processes that serve to maintain the problem. In Translating Predisposing, Precipitating, and Perpetuating Aspects of Risk Into Prevention and Treatment, we describe how the mechanisms that underpin eating problems in a patient can be used to plan the form of treatment.

Translating Predisposing, Precipitating, and Perpetuating Aspects of Risk into Prevention and Treatment

Tailoring Treatment to Predisposing Factors

In this section, we discuss the environmental, social, and developmental factors that interplay and lead to the development of an ED and suggest how those can be targeted in treatment.

Environmental Factors

Cultural predisposing factors include easy access to palatable food, loss of meal structure, and social eating, and idealisation of thinness. Cultural factors are of particular relevance to binge EDs. A focus of behaviour change in therapy is, therefore, to target the patterns of eating that become disrupted in these disorders. The aim, therefore, is to plan regular meals that contain a sufficient quantity and quality of food to meet nutritional needs.

Target Behaviour: The Culture of Eating

- Introduce a regular pattern of eating meals containing natural basic foods that have not been highly processed and have a low glycaemic index.
- Ensure that there is a nutritional balance of the macronutrients (protein, fat, carbohydrates) and micronutrients (vitamins and minerals).
- Use strategies to decrease habits related to access and consumption of high-fat/high-sugar foods.
- Embed meals into a social matrix.

In contemporary culture, there are both aesthetic and health concerns about overweight. The focus within therapy or prevention is to question the reality, feasibility, and health aspects of some of the extremes portrayed in fashion and media. Improving media literacy to enable critical appraisal of fashion images is a helpful component of many prevention programmes. The use of dissonance-based techniques, whereby the individual proposes arguments to counteract the thinness ideal, is helpful. Body image work in treatment uses behavioural experiments to counteract dysfunctional behaviours, such as checking and avoidance of body exposure-related experiences. Second, widening the horizon of meaningful life values beyond those related to the body, an aesthetic object, to the broader aspects of human beings as functioning units in society, is a key focus in therapy. This includes issues such as the values associated with identity, citizenship, and civilisation.

Target Behaviour: The Culture of Thinness

- Question media portrayals of thinness.
- Use a broad focus on values, identity, and citizenship.
- Focus on positive aspects of body. Emphasise the body in action and function, rather than a static object of observation.
- Eliminate dysfunctional behaviours, such as body checking and avoidance.

Predisposing Factors from the Perinatal Environment

Stress and nutritional factors within the perinatal environment can have profound and persistent effects on physiology and psychology. Exposure to stress during the perinatal period can produce an overactive hypothalamic–pituitary–adrenal axis. This heightened stress sensitivity can be moderated by antidepressants and a safe, secure environment with strong interpersonal attachments and careful planning and preparation for transitions. A strong therapeutic alliance can be a cornerstone for change.

Target Behaviour: Overactive Hypothalamic–Pituitary–Adrenal Axis

- Antidepressants to decrease overactivity of the hypothalamic–pituitary–adrenal axis.
- Strong attachments and planning to take 'safe' risks.

Nutritional factors in the perinatal period can negatively affect metabolism, blood pressure, and other physiological factors throughout life. Individuals exposed to malnutrition during the perinatal period will need a broad-based healthy lifestyle.

Target Behaviour: A Predisposition to Obesity and Cardiovascular Risk

- Lifestyle factors to moderate risk include exercise, healthy eating, and a balance of life rhythms, with regular periods set aside for sleep, eating, work and relaxation.

Family and Peer Predisposing Factors: Food and Weight Salience, Parental Weight, Teasing, and Criticism – 'Shapeism'

Within the family or the local peer environment, there may be a particular salience ascribed to weight and shape issues, above and beyond what is normal in that culture. This may relate to the attitudes toward food within the family, including both cryptic and overt EDs within the family. Teasing, criticism, or comments about weight and shape, and eating within the family, is a particularly potent risk factor. Certain sports or careers may promote or demand specific body characteristics, which may or may not be attainable.

Target Behaviour: Overvaluation of Food, Weight, or Shape within the Family or Peer Group

- Exploration of attitudes within the family and peer group with moderation of expressed emotion (criticism, hostility, overprotection) about these issues.

Precipitating Life Events

An aim of therapy is to strengthen resilience with robust emotional regulation and coping strategies to life events. This includes improving problem solving, practical and emotional coping, and decreasing maladaptive coping, such as avoidance, rumination, not eating, and compulsive exercise. There is also a focus on predisposing personality traits, such as intolerance of uncertainty, perfectionism and rigidity that may be linked to unhelpful metacognitive poor coping strategies. The aim is to foster adaptive emotional regulation strategies (awareness of emotions and adaptive use of emotions to guide behaviours) rather than experiential avoidance. The focus is turned toward positive aspects of life rather than dwelling on the negative aspects and cognitive reappraisal is a key tool.

Target Behaviour: Maladaptive Coping Strategies

- Optimistic attitude – elicit strengths and positive values of the individual by using a solution focused or a motivational interviewing style of interaction.
- Reduce avoidance – encourage approaching in the form of behavioural experiments.
- Increase emotional intelligence with the wise use of emotions to inform behaviours. Teach emotional literacy, what is the body felt sense, and what need is the emotion signalling.
- Reduce inappropriately high, unrealistic standards.
- Increase focus on the big picture – a well-lived life rather than a focus on the detail of minor imperfections.
- Increase flexibility – add in small change steps to foster brain plasticity.
- Increase attachment to the world and others.

Genetic Risk Factors: Anomalies in the Control of Appetite, Reward, and Stress

This strategy involves adapting the environment to moderate genetic extremes. Here, there is overlap with dispositions that are thought to arise as a result of an interaction between genetic and environmental factors (see Target Behaviour: Anomalies in Appetite, Reward, and Stress Systems).

Target Behaviour: Anomalies in Appetite, Reward, and Stress Systems

- The use of regular exercise and healthy diet to moderate the impact of thrifty genes (relevant for binge eating).
- Diversification of pleasant aspects of life.
- Buffer a sensitivity to stress by encouraging a sense of safety through connection with others and consider antidepressants.

Predisposing Risk Factors: Anxiety, Obsessive–Compulsive Personality Disorder Traits, Low Self-Esteem, Poor Social Aptitude

Many of the developmental predisposing risk factors emerge from either genetic or environmental factors, or an interaction between the two. A focus of therapy is to remediate these traits and help individuals to move away from extremes. This process involves procedures such as feedback, retraining to allow focus on the underdeveloped pole, and to provide balance. For example, cognitive remediation followed by training is used to increase flexibility and to be able to step back to see the bigger picture.

Emotional training is used to focus on positive emotions and to buffer negative emotions with empathy and compassion (for the self and others). This process will help to improve social cognition and social relationships. Encourage developing a diverse range of social connection (choir, yoga, ecology, etc.). The aim is to strengthen a positive self-image and decrease emotional avoidance strategies self-harm or starvation.

Target Behaviour: Anomalies in Predisposing Behaviour – Rigidity, Excess Detail, Anxiety, and Low Self-Esteem

- Train emotional intelligence.
- Train to develop a positive and compassionate attitude toward self and others.
- Consider antidepressants to reduce dysregulated stress.
- Consider antipsychotics to reduce the strength of the anorexic voice in anorexia nervosa (AN).
- Strengthen attachments to provide security.
- Train flexibility and bigger picture thinking.
- Use behavioural experiments to use different ways to cope.
- Focus on positive aspects of body as actor versus object.
- Increase social connection.
- Train media literacy.

Tailoring Treatment to Perpetuating or Maintaining Factors

In addition to these predisposing risk factors, the main focus of treatment is on the maintaining factors. It is particularly helpful to focus on the maintaining factors within treatment because, by definition, these are present in current behaviours and so provide the opportunity to be modified. Some of the dispositions that are risk factors, such as rigidity, a focus on detail, and poor emotional regulation, tend to be accentuated by starvation, and act to perpetuate the illness.

Maintaining Factors for AN

One of the reasons that people with AN are of two minds about change is that there are many positive consequences that arise from the illness, and match with their personality or coping style. These obviously vary between individuals, but some examples include eliciting care and concern from others, an excuse for failing at overly high standards, loss of menstrual periods and interest in sexuality, and loss of emotional reactivity. The process of motivational enhancement therapy includes an exploration of ambivalence about change with both written and verbal tasks that focus on possible secondary gains. The aim is to help find other means to attain these positive consequences of the ED.

The interpersonal reactions that are thought to perpetuate AN include carers responding with high expressed emotion (overprotection or criticism), inadvertently rewarding ED behaviours, and not attending to non-ED behaviours. Families benefit from being given skills and information about interpersonal reactions, to help them understand and manage the illness. This can be delivered in the form of guided self-care, group, or individual sessions (see Chapter 11).

Social cognition decreases with weight loss. This disturbs interpersonal behaviour as mirroring and emotional reciprocity is reduced.

Obsessive–compulsive traits such as perfectionism, inflexibility, preoccupation with detail, and intolerance of uncertainty become more pronounced once the illness starts. Once these traits are fixed onto the goal of weight loss, they serve to provide effective strategies for further weight loss.

Target Behaviour: Maintaining Factors for AN

- Explore the positive aspects of AN and develop more adaptive behaviours to meet these goals.
- Emotion and skills training for close others (and the individual) to moderate interpersonal reactions that develop with AN.
- Obsessive–compulsive traits such as rigidity and a narrow detailed focus by encouraging flexibility and bigger picture thinking.
- The development of a compassionate stance to moderate anxiety, social submission, and avoidance behaviours.
- Decrease social isolation by developing a large social network.

Maintaining Factors for Bulimia Nervosa

The avoidance behaviours related to food such as prolonged fasting, the omission of social eating, and strict dietary rules serve to perpetuate bulimia nervosa (BN). In addition, methods used to avoid weight gain such as purging serve to increase both the physiological as well the psychological drivers of food craving. A main focus of treatment is to reverse these avoidance behaviours by reintroducing a planned structure to meals. The use of food diaries to structure and monitor eating behaviours is an important component of treatment. In addition, education and experiments to moderate the cognitions that underpin the unhelpful use of avoidance strategies is a key component. This can be done by interrupting body checking, for example.

The increase in reward sensitivity means that more attention is focused on food cues and the sense of deprivation in the withdrawal state becomes more painful. Strategies to reduce the increased salience of binge foods include managing exposure to shops, buffets, and other food stores. Planning in which healthy habits are cued by environmental triggers (implementation intentions) followed by reflection can decrease the impulsive urge to act when craving starts. Monitoring awareness using food diaries (perhaps photographing food to be eaten) and limiting exposure are helpful. The process of craving can be disrupted, using distraction, acceptance, and mindfulness strategies. The dysphoric state can be managed with antidepressants or adaptive emotional regulation strategies.

Once a binge occurs, the overconsumption of food leads to regret and anxiety about having broken the strict dietary rules. An attempt of reparation for this lapse then follows, using a variety of reversing behaviours (fasting, vomiting, laxatives, etc). However, those methods that prevent the absorption of food in turn exacerbate the sense of deprivation, which leads to more craving and a predisposition to overeat, and the cycle starts again. The maintaining factors come into play.

Target Behaviour: Maintaining Factors for BN

- Focus on normalising the pattern, context, and content of eating by reversing ED habits by planning and monitoring food behaviours.
- Interrupt reversing behaviours (e.g., purging, fasting, and exercise) by planning and monitoring.
- Teach strategies to moderate the salience of food cues (e.g., shopping lists and reduce hunger).
- Increase social connection and activity to have a wider range of rewarding activity.

Maintaining Factors for Binge EDs

The first phase of treatment includes an explanation about the psychology and physiology of eating described in Chapter 2. A description of maintaining factors for binge eating are then discussed. These overlap with the features described for BN.

- Teach emotional regulation strategies e.g. acceptance and management of emotional states.

The Processes Needed for Behaviour Change

A common element across all of the EDs is the need to change behaviours. Of course, the obvious first behaviour that needs changing is eating. However, depending on the formulation, there are many other areas in which behaviour change is needed; for example, improved communication, assertiveness, social engagement, flexibility, and global perspective taking. The order in which to prioritise these goals is a matter of clinical judgement and depends on the level of risk, perceived difficulty, and personal preference.

A focus on the changes required to alleviate high medical risk is essential. However, if therapy is stuck in terms of weight gain and no acute medical risk exists, moving onto another therapeutic goal can sidestep resistance. Similarly, if one behaviour change process does not seem to work, try another. A key element in therapy is to be flexible and to keep a good warm therapeutic relationship alive. Table 12.1 lists the elements of behaviour change processes that have been found to be of use for people with EDs. Many of these elements form the core of cognitive behaviour therapy for BN.

Outline of the Processes Used in the Management of EDs

The Form of Therapy

Interpersonal issues form a key aspect of both the aetiology and maintenance of EDs. This has implications for the therapeutic relationship, the content of therapy, and who is involved in treatment.

The Therapeutic Relationship

The key issue in treatment is engagement in the therapeutic relationship. This issue is particularly problematic for people with AN. Using the terminology of the transtheoretical model of change, most patients are in precontemplation, not ready to change, or contemplation in two minds about change. The strategies of motivational interviewing can facilitate movement into action by increasing the importance and confidence that an improvement in nutritional health is necessary.

The clinician should have a compassionate, empathetic stance. Confrontation and a dominating response is unhelpful. The therapist needs to be gentle and kind. The voice (soft and soothing) and body posture (signifying listening and cooperation) are part of the process as much as words. The key aspects of motivational interviewing include rolling with resistance (avoiding confrontation), developing discrepancy (eliciting pros and cons of change), supporting self-efficacy (encouraging autonomy), and expressing empathy (mnemonic RR, DD, SS, and EE) are invaluable. Open questions, affirmations, reflections and summaries keep the process in motion.

Table 12.1 Elements of behaviour change processes of use for people with EDs

Step	Element	Actions
1	Medical monitoring and feedback	Weight (each session). Short physical examination, BP (lie and stand), pulse rate, temperature, myopathy, peripheral circulation including oedema and laboratory tests) – frequency determined by risk. The frequency of other tests depends on clinical judgement (see medical risk chart, www.eatingresearch.com) and Chapters 4, 5, 6, and 11.
2	General information on the behaviour–health link	Review of the life domains that are impacted by an ED (medical, psychological, social (family), education/career, citizen, spiritual).
3	Information on consequences	Benefits and costs of change versus no change. Expand on the long-term consequences regarding the costs of no change. The individual is encouraged to step back from the here and now to review their life as a whole. (We have termed this the Christmas Carol approach as we invoke reflection upon ghosts of the past and future with and without an ED.)
4	Provide information about the concern of others	Involve family members or close others in the assessment (with a face-to-face or virtual meeting). (This will depend on the potential impact on others, which in turn depends on age, level of dependence, and risk.) This session needs to be carefully managed to ensure that there is an emphasis on approval and acknowledgement for non-ED behaviour and change efforts, rather than merely an opportunity for criticism of the ED. Provide education for the family so that they have more understanding of the illness and are able to manage their own unhelpful emotional reactions relating to the illness (e.g., the elements of high expressed emotion, criticism, and overprotection).
5	Prompt formation of intentions	Encourage the individual to make a behavioural resolution. The domain to be changed will depend on level of risk and the formulation
		Typical goals relating to food and meals include eating a sufficient amount with a nutritionally balanced content, meals that are spaced at intervals within the day, and meals tied into social conventions. In addition to food, there may be goals relating to other maintaining factors such as obsessive–compulsive traits. Goals in this case may include increased flexibility and bigger picture thinking. Emotion-processing goals include improving awareness and regulation. Interpersonal goals include decreasing isolation and increasing cooperation, trust and engagement with core values,
6	Prompt barrier identification	Spend time planning how to overcome potential barriers such as competing goals (e.g., avoiding anxiety). This may involve problem solving and skills training related to goals as described in step 5.

Table 12.1 *(cont.)*

7	Provide general encouragement	Give affirmations for effort in the process of change, rather than praise contingent on narrowly defined behavioural performance. The latter can seem patronising and can also invoke past experiences of contingent care and affection.
8	Set graded tasks	Set easy to perform tasks in the first instance and gradually make them more difficult.
9	Model/demonstrate behaviour	This can include eating or skills relating to other goals, e.g., communication and emotional expression.
10	Prompt specific goal setting	Make a detailed proposal with goal setting including frequency, intensity, and duration of the planned behaviours. Meticulous specification of the context such as where, when, how, or with whom and including subgoals, and preparatory behaviours. In some cases, this will involve the use of imagery
11	Prompt review of behaviour goal	Weigh each session for patients with AN. Reflect on other food-related goals such as the frequency of binges or normal meals and compensatory behaviours.
12	Prompt self-monitoring of behaviour	Display a weight chart, for example. Diaries monitoring food/meal goals and compensatory behaviours.
13	Provide feedback on performance	This should include reflection on achievements in step 11 and identifying discrepancies with expressed intention (step 4) and specific goal planning (step 10).
14	Provide contingent rewards	For the most part, this will be praise and encouragement, although for the inpatient treatment of AN it can involve more concrete rewards (time out, etc.) if the planned behaviour change is completed.
15	Teach to use prompts/cues	Identify environmental prompts as a reminder to perform behaviour (e.g., text from friend at meal times) or other aspects of the context that can cue exhibiting or inhibiting the target behaviour.
16	Contract of behavioural agreement	This is often used in care planning on inpatient settings. It involves a written record of person's resolution witnessed by another.
17	Prompt practice	This may relate to some of the goals set.
18	Use of follow-up prompts	This involves some contact by phone, email, letters, or follow-up meetings.
19	Provide opportunities for social comparison	Indirectly, this is a component of the assessment and feedback process and involves the objective presentation of individual data alongside normative data, e.g., presenting the individual's weight on a BMI chart. The results of medical tests, e.g., blood workup and neuropsychiatric tests, can be used in this way. In addition, this can be a component of

Table 12.1 *(cont.)*

		behavioural experiments in which an individual will compare herself objectively with healthy individuals. Inpatient or group settings provide direct opportunities for this.
20	Plan social support/ social change	This involves prompting the individual to think about how others could change their behaviour to offer help and instrumental social support. This can be negotiated in family meetings. It may include help reducing ED behaviour or increasing non-ED behaviour. It can be helpful for family members to be involved in goal setting and implementing behaviour change techniques when the individual is at the stage where they are ready to make changes. Family members may need to acquire the skills to manage a situation in which there is a tension between their goals and those of the individual who might remain highly ambivalent about change. The support network may need the skills of motivational interviewing to manage this mixed agenda (step 25).
21	Prompt self-identification as role model/position advocate	Elicit strategies from them by asking them to visualise talking to others about changing their behaviour. Also provide opportunities for participants to think about preventing others from taking up the behaviour (possibly a written task), e.g., if they had a daughter, what would they do to prevent her developing an ED?
22	Prompt self-talk	Encourage the person to talk to themselves (aloud or silently) before and during planned behaviours to encourage and support action. (Encouraging self-talk about change within the session is a key element in motivation interviewing; step 25).
23	Relapse prevention	Following on from initial changes, help the person to identify situations that increase the likelihood of problem behaviour returning. Help plan how to avoid or manage the situation so that new behaviours are maintained.
24	Stress management	Teach a variety of specific techniques, e.g., progressive relaxation, guided imagery, etc., which reduce arousal. In addition, this may include emotion control training to reduce emotional upset or control moods and feelings which interfere with change. An additional technique is to encourage written reflections to produce a multidimensional account of emotional awareness (essays, letters from different perspectives – time, person, etc.). These types of approaches are exemplified in dialectical behaviour therapy, acceptance and commitment therapy, emotional-focused therapy.
25	MI	This communication style is designed to elicit talk about change from individuals who are not fully willing or able to consider change. It is particularly useful for individuals with AN who are the most ambivalent about change. However, it can be used when there is resistance to any aspect of goal

Table 12.1 (*cont.*)

	planning; e.g., individuals with BN are often resistant to planning to eat regularly. This style includes the use of open questions, reflections, affirmations, and summaries and has a directive element by eliciting and reinforcing the individuals talking and planning for change. Motivational enhancement is an extension of MI. It involves looking at consequences (step 2) and prompts anticipated regret (how an individual will feel in the future and whether they will feel sorry that they did not take a different course). It also aims to increase self-efficacy about change by prompting a focus on past success (i.e., thinking about previous success in changing target or allied behaviours.

Abbreviations: AN, anorexia nervosa; BN, bulimia nervosa; BP, blood pressure; ED, eating disorder; MI, motivational interviewing.

Thus, the first phase of engagement with patients with and ED is a period of motivational interviewing to explore who wants treatment (usually family, doctors, and tutors are the prime movers) and why (move onto the overall quality of the patient's life). Once a good therapeutic alliance is established, it is possible to get some commitment to behaviour change.

The Interpersonal Content of Therapy

People with AN have a variety of problems in social and emotional function. They judge themselves as inferior to others and undertake a variety of submissive behaviours (appeasing powerful others) or striving to stave off feelings of inferiority. This focus is key to their therapy. In addition, people with EDs have problems with emotional recognition, processing, regulation, and communication. Work with close others can target some of these difficulties.

The Involvement of the Family in the Management of AN

AN is a highly visible disorder. Commonly, AN elicits a caregiving response that can promote the sick role and infantilise the individual. An unintended consequence is that overprotection leads to a failure to develop mastery, self-confidence, and self-esteem. Families can sometimes allow themselves to be bullied by the person with the ED and accommodate and accept the behaviours or even play a role in them. Another common response from the family is frustration and anger that the patient refuses to do what they 'should' do, i.e., eat. This criticism and hostility increases anxiety and alienation, which in turn increases ED behaviour.

Aside from these direct effects, which are more common when families are living together, having a relative with a chronic, life-threatening illness is stressful. Families express a need for information and help. Group educational interventions for family members have been found to decrease the distress, expressed emotion, and caregiving burden and are highly valued by the families. There is some evidence that patient outcomes are also improved.

The involvement of families in treatment depends on several factors: the age of the patient, living arrangements, the level of risk and dependence, and the ethos of the treatment team.

Conclusion

In this chapter, we have discussed some of the components that are required in the treatment of an ED. An illustration of how these modules can interact and need to be integrated for AN is shown in Figure 13.1. Engagement, motivation, and risk assessment are the essential initial platform from which all other components are built. The exploration and remediation of the risk and maintaining factors may be facilitated by the inclusion of close others in treatment.

Implications for Health Care Professionals

- The 'brand name' of any therapy used for the management of AN is probably less important than the form (what sort of therapeutic relationship – collaborative with high empathy and low dominance) and the content (behaviour change processes targeting aspects of the formulation).
- Developing a good therapeutic alliance is essential in the management of ED, particularly AN.
- The therapist has to be flexible and sensitive to recognise which behaviour to focus on and how, when, and with what process to do so.
- Developing a formulation with an emphasis on precipitating, predisposing and perpetuating factors is an important template for treatment and can also provide meaning.

Diabetes Mellitus

Case

A 19-year-old woman with type 1 diabetes mellitus presents with confusion, depression, and disordered eating.

Comment

People with type 1 diabetes have an increased risk of developing all forms of EDs. There are several reasons that may account for this such as the salience of weight and eating in this condition and the difficulties of living with a chronic illness. The following are possible mechanisms:

1. Weight fluxes are often present in type 1 diabetes. Weight loss is common in the prodromal phase because glucose is lost in the urine. Treatment with insulin can lead to a rapid increase in weight as a result of rehydration and replenishment of glycogen stores. Patients therefore can associate insulin treatment with an increase in 'fat' and hence to use insulin omission as a means of avoiding weight gain.
2. The treatment of diabetes has a focus on food, eating, and weight.
3. Living with a chronic illness can decrease self-esteem. Social anxiety and shame may result from the complex and intrusive self-management procedures.
4. Recent genetic findings suggest that there are metabolic vulnerabilities in EDs.

The core treatment of type 1 diabetes mellitus is based on specialised diabetic education and management to adjust insulin administration to ensure that blood glucose falls within the normal range. (There are now novel automated advances that are being introduced.) Feedback about the success of this replacement regime is obtained by regular blood glucose readings and blood tests (glycosylated haemoglobin).

People with type 1 diabetes and an ED have difficulties following the treatment plan. They avoid routine appointments but may be admitted with diabetic ketoacidosis or other complications (see Table 12.1).

Complications of Diabetes Mellitus Worsened by an ED

- Metabolic: hypoglycaemia causing loss of consciousness, ketoacidosis causing reduced level of consciousness.
- Small vessels: retinopathy, renal failure, reduced blood supply to the skin.
- Large vessels: stroke, heart attack, peripheral vascular disease, renal artery disease.
- Infection: increase chance of bacterial infection, infection of feet and legs can progress rapidly requiring amputation.

These patients also respond poorly to standard ED treatment. Treatment guidelines recommend forms of joint management between medical and psychosocial care. However, it is important that there is integration and cooperation and a shared ethos between these components. Some aspects of treatments might be seen to clash. For example, one component of ED treatment is to decrease rule-driven eating and to encourage a more regular, intuitive pattern of eating. The contrasts with the success of diabetes educational interventions such as DAPHNE, which involves careful rules and planning.

In addition, perfectionism is a risk and maintaining factor for EDs. Overly high expectations (from self and possibly diabetic staff) may be counterproductive in the context of the complexities of diabetes management. The sense of failure from not meeting 'perfect glucose control' can be dispiriting and demotivating. Appetite and metabolic systems are complex, and genetic vulnerabilities may add to the difficulties in obtaining normal levels of glucose. Furthermore, the strategies needed to attain 'control' are intrusive and socially disruptive. Interventions for ED aim to moderate perfectionistic goals and hence shift the glucose goal from excellent to 'good enough', which may seem to run counter to what they perceive that the diabetic team want.

Judgmental words such as good and bad, glucose levels/food, and the use of the word control should avoided because these patients are sensitised to social criticism. Therefore, a collaborative model of care is needed, including friends and family to avoid cultural clashes, which may lead to a lack of trust and withdrawal from treatment. Such a cooperative approach requires members of the diabetic team to use psychotherapeutic skills. Furthermore, inpatient ED teams need expertise to provide tailored diabetic care for these patients. For example, the reintroduction of insulin can be accompanied by extreme oedema. These weight changes reinforce the terror that insulin produces fatness. Also, treatment-related complications (neuropathy) can result from producing too rapid a restoration of normal sugar levels from a baseline of persistent hyperglycaemia. The extreme fear and aversion to insulin treatment may be overcome by a gradual titration of insulin with a diet low in carbohydrates in the initial phase.

Management of Diabetes Mellitus in Patients with an ED

- Education: Both general diabetes education and specific diabetic/ED education are needed. This may include how to incorporate stress management techniques such as regular exercise ideally in a social context.
- Diet: An initial phase with a low carbohydrate diet can be a helpful adaption that can decrease the need for insulin in the initial exposure phase.
- Monitoring: Ideally, regular blood sugar monitoring is needed (it is possible for this to be automated).
- Insulin: The insulin regimen should be managed by agreement between the patient and the diabetic specialist. Insulin pump treatment may facilitate management.

Implications for Health Care Professionals on an Inpatient Unit

- Supervise blood glucose monitoring and recording.
- Supervise insulin administration.
- Have regular diabetic reviews and liaison.

Shoplifting

Case

Your patient tells you, 'I'm just tired of alternating my eating disorder with my shoplifting because I cannot deal with my feelings of guilt, shame, anger, and fear.' She asks you whether other patients with an ED shoplift and whether you can help her.

Comment

Shoplifting can lead to a criminal conviction and record, which can make it impossible to be bonded, qualify for certain jobs, or visit or work in some countries. For a young person, these repercussions are serious. This information may motivate a patient to provide a more complete history of shoplifting behaviour and seek treatment.

Shoplifting is more common in patients with an ED than in controls. Among patients with an ED, it is more common in those who binge and purge than those who do not. We reported a life-time prevalence of one episode of shoplifting in 56 per cent of those with AN with bingeing/purging, 52 per cent of those with BN, 50 per cent of ED not otherwise specified, and 36 per cent of those with the AN restricting subtype, and more frequent shoplifting in 19 per cent of those with BN, 14 per cent of those with AN with bingeing/purging, 9 per cent of those with the AN restricting subtype, and 7 per cent of those with ED not otherwise specified. Patients who shoplift regularly are likely to steal food and the belongings of others in hospital or as an outpatient. This situation causes an ethical dilemma; how to maintain confidentiality, while not increasing the risk of the patient stealing, and protecting the belongings of others. This dilemma should be dealt with on a case-by-case basis. Refusing treatment based on a history of shoplifting is unethical.

Behavioural therapy; cognitive–behavioural therapy; pharmacological treatment with mood stabilisers, selective serotonin reuptake inhibitors, and opioid receptor antagonists;

and twelve-step groups may be effective for some patients. Therapy should be individualised. A letter to the judge stating that the patient is being treated for an ED, and that shoplifting is associated with EDs, may result in a single reprieve.

Implications for Health Care Professionals

- Take a history of shoplifting behaviour; it is common, especially in those who binge and purge, and it will not be volunteered.
- Inform the patient that shoplifting can lead to a criminal conviction and a criminal record. This can make it impossible to be bonded, qualify for certain jobs, or visit or work in some countries.
- Encourage the patient to begin therapy for shoplifting.
- Decide with your colleagues, and with the patient, how you will manage the risk of stealing, before the admission.

Substance Use

Case

A 23-year-old woman is referred to you for treatment of AN, bingeing/purging subtype. She describes daily use of crystal methamphetamine to control her appetite and monthly binge use, staying awake for up to 3 days at time. She has been admitted previously to an intensive residential addiction treatment program, but was discharged prematurely because she could not control her purging.

Comment

Substance use disorders occur with increased frequency in patients with EDs. The strength of the relationship between these disorders varies considerably. In part, this varies with the populations studied and how substance use and disordered eating are defined. The strength of association is strongest in patients with BN and binge ED, weaker in patients with ED not otherwise specified and AN purging type, and not considered significant in patients with restricting AN. There is the suggestion that disorders with loss of control over eating may be underpinned by addictive brain changes, which may account for this increased risk. This may explain why patient with EDs can experience more negative consequences from substance use compared with substance use patients without EDs.

Effect of Substance Use on Patients with EDs

People use substances for a variety of reasons, but there are specific pharmacological reasons why patients with EDs may use substances. Psychostimulants such as cocaine, amphetamines, and ecstasy suppress appetite and increase the metabolic rate, generally resulting in weight loss with regular use. Nicotine also suppresses appetite and increases metabolic rate, resulting in more modest weight loss with regular use. Conversely, marijuana stimulates appetite and may be used by patients with EDs to decrease anxiety around food and eating, generally resulting in weight gain with regular use. Alcohol in sufficient dosage suppresses appetite, but its effect on weight is variable because alcohol itself is a source of calories, and may also be used by patients with EDs to decrease anxiety around food and eating, thereby increasing food intake.

Substance use and dependence results in neglect of activities that are not related to substance use such as procurement, preparation, and consumption of food, placing all patients with substance use disorders at risk for malnutrition and weight loss. The risk is obviously heightened in patients with EDs. Furthermore, chronic use of substances such as alcohol places patients at increased risk for specific nutritional deficiencies, such as deficiencies of thiamine, folate, vitamin B_{12}, and magnesium.

Substance intoxication and withdrawal states are often associated with loss of appetite, nausea, vomiting, or diarrhoea. Patients with EDs in these states may therefore have an increased risk of volume depletion, electrolyte disorders, and arrhythmias.

The circumstances in which substances are consumed (e.g., binge consumption, rave parties) may also place patients with EDs at increased risk for volume depletion, electrolyte disorders, and arrhythmias.

Substance use increases the risk of suicide. This is relevant for all patients with mental disorders.

Substance use disorders may interfere with a patient's ability to attend follow-up appointments, cooperate with hospitalisation or refeeding, or participate in residential treatment programmes.

Treatment Models

In the past, ED treatment programmes often excluded patients with active substance use disorders. Such patients were referred to addiction treatment programmes to have that problem treated before entering into ED treatment. This 'in-series treatment' model is problematic because it is often impossible to determine which disorder should be treated first, and both disorders are associated with a high rate of relapse after treatment. In this model, the patient frequently bounces back and forth between the two treatment systems. The ED impairs the patient's ability to complete treatment for the substance use disorder and vice versa.

More recently, a 'parallel treatment' model has been used. In this model, both disorders are treated at the same time by different treatment systems. This model is an improvement, but remains problematic because there is often little communication between the two treatment systems and patients are often given conflicting recommendations. It is hoped that the introduction of the food addiction model as part of treatment will allow for a more coherent approach.

An 'integrated treatment' model, where both disorders are treated concurrently in the same system is thought to represent the ideal way to treat patients with substance use disorders and any mental illness, including EDs. EDs and addiction treatment programmes must strive to create such models.

Implications for Health Care Professionals

- Screen all patients for substance use disorders.
- Look for signs and symptoms of substance intoxication and withdrawal in all patients admitted to ED treatment programmes.
- Develop treatment models and policies that support the integrated treatment of EDs and substance use disorders.

The Chronic Patient

Case

Cindy was a 40-year-old woman with AN who I had followed for 20 years, until her death. She had severe, unremitting, restrictive AN complicated by hyponatremia, hypokalaemia, hypomagnesemia, an empyema of her lung, multiple bone fractures, renal failure, anaemia, and, terminally, pneumonia and acute inferior myocardial infarction. Cindy had been admitted repeatedly over the years to various ED units. She had tried and given up on many psychiatrists and psychologists, she was on chronic disability leave from her work, and a few years before her death she moved to an apartment in a suburb where she would eat very small amounts of food and have intermittent infusions of saline, potassium, and magnesium in her home. Cindy had been emaciated for years, but she enjoyed helping others and always asked me about my children and would send them birthday presents. Although she could hardly hobble around with the use of her cane, she dressed in vividly coloured clothes and maintained her dignity to the end.

Comment

The treatment of patients with chronic AN is widely misunderstood. As in many illnesses, the rate of recovery is variable. The average patient with AN may have the disorder for a few years, but many patients will continue to be anorexic for many years and some for life. Many health professionals feel guilty and confused when it seems that treatment does not work. Many patients are told that 'nothing else can be done' and discharged from care, without arranging any alternative treatment. Those who continue to follow the patients with chronic AN often consciously adopt a palliative care approach to the treatment of patients with 'chronic' AN, where palliative means treatment of discomfort but nothing else. This is tantamount to providing only palliative care to a patient who continues to present with asthma attacks.

In chronic AN, the treatment approach should be a chronic disease or rehabilitative approach, rather than a palliative approach. This approach shifts the goal of treatment from cure to quality of life.

- Treatment of intercurrent medical and psychiatric conditions continues.
- Focus treatment goals on quality of life through rehabilitation
- Continue to treat malnutrition, limited by the patient's goals.
- The patient may choose to begin standard treatment at any time.

Remission in chronic AN may occur after a life-changing event (e.g., divorce, death of a parent, deciding to change carriers) or when then patient can no longer tolerate being burdened with the disease. All patients can recover from AN; some recover decades into their illness. The health care professional must adopt the chronic disease or rehabilitation model, not the palliative model, for patients who suffer from chronic AN

Patients with chronic AN have ongoing signs and symptoms of protein–calorie malnutrition. They will have thinning of their hair, dry and yellow skin, a decreased ability to focus their eyes, shortness of breath on exertion, decreased exercise capacity, repeated arrhythmias, dizziness on standing, weakness, tiredness, hypothermia, muscle cramps, and decreased memory and concentration. In addition, they will suffer from progressive osteopenia, which will cause repeated fractures; these begin as stress factors and later become fractures of the spine and lower extremities.

Chronic AN is associated with social isolation, an inability to work and learn, and diminished functional activity, including with family, friends, and at work. Depending on the level of debilitation, the patient may be reclusive, living in a small apartment and isolated from their family, or they may be a thin individual with significant weight and shape concerns who is fully integrated into their family, work, and society. Clearly, the goal of rehabilitation is to move a patient with AN from the former to the latter situation.

Goals When Following the Chronic Patient

- Prevent death by monitoring depression, actively preventing suicide, building rapport, searching for psychological comorbidity that might prevent improvement or diminish quality of life, helping to set goals for rehabilitation, and continuing to celebrate life with the patient at every visit.
- Medically, the frequency of follow-up varies, depending on the degree of illness, from every week to every 3 months. The weight, blood pressure, and heart rate should be measured. An inquiry regarding mood and plans should be taken, and goals should be established. If the patient is losing or gaining weight, then measure potassium, magnesium, and phosphate. If the weight is unchanged, this is not necessary. If there is significant deterioration in physical symptoms, a systemic inquiry and physical examination with laboratory measures selected based on symptoms (often hemoglobin, electrolytes, creatinine, AST, alkaline phosphatase, magnesium, phosphate, vitamin B_{12}, and ferritin) should be performed.

The physician should concentrate first on physical complaints. Chronic anorexics find it much easier to talk about physical concerns. Treatment of physical problems is easily accepted and appreciated, and this increases rapport. Treatment of urinary incontinence (which commonly occurs in chronic AN), careful care of feet and toes, and prevention of osteopenia with calcium and vitamin D supplements should all be considered. Use of the birth control pill to continue menstruation or for contraception can be discussed, but it is not effective as a treatment for osteoporosis.

Psychologically, focus on rehabilitation and quality of life. Any comorbid condition, such as a history of sexual abuse, substance use, or depression, should be sought and may require long-term treatment before other psychological gains are possible. Patients should be encouraged to attend motivational enhancement therapy.

The family doctor may find the narrative approach useful when setting goals. This approach helps to set goals by encouraging the patient to tell the story of their life over the next few years, as if they were looking back in time from the future. They are 'writing the story of their life'. The issues of eating, weight, and shape are not discussed. The narrative approach should focus in particular on what would make their story satisfying or exciting to them. Often, it is useful to refocus the patient on their life by pretending it is a movie and changing the ending or episodes of the movie as they would if they were directing it.

One must be very careful regarding the involvement of the family in the treatment of chronic AN. Other family members may hold powerful feelings of guilt and anger toward the anorexic. The anorexic patient may also be ostracised from their family. Therefore, any discussions with the family members are best done at the patient's request and with the patient present. As a primary physician, these often are in the form of family interventions. For example, the patient may wish to change their place of residence, apply for disability insurance, or discuss their position in the family. A physician can act as a mediator for the patient and explain the patient's disease in the context of a process for which chronic rehabilitation is necessary. It is of immense importance that the primary physician respect the right of privacy of the patient. This is particularly difficult in the setting of a family physician who has treated the entire family for years. All patients who reach the age of majority should be treated as independent adults – regardless of their health or place of residence. All parties – the patient, their family, and other hospital staff – must be aware of this policy; otherwise, confidentiality will likely be breached and the patient's trust lost forever.

Medically, there are no medications other than food that are of absolute necessity in chronic AN. Some patients will accept ciproheptadine, which can be given at a dose of 4–16 mg at bedtime to increase fatty mass somewhat.

Exercise is useful in AN. Our work in the use of yoga in-hospital and with a graded exercise program out-of-hospital to focus on breathing, stretching and gradual incorporation of exercise to try to increase lean body mass and maintain bony mass is gaining acceptance. Paradoxically, exercise may decrease with a very gradual introduction of minimal activity in the patient with chronic AN. Certainly if the physician simply proscribes activity, this is likely not to be accepted by the patient.

Implications for Health Care Professionals

- Treat specific complaints, such as osteoporosis, chronic pain, and depression.
- Improve their quality of life: weakness or other complaints that reduce quality of life should be investigated and treated. Treatment should be based on a rehabilitation approach.
- Motivation to change: during the course of the disease, many chronic patients will ask to engage in active therapy for their AN. This should be recognised and treated as a great opportunity.

Chapter 13

Medical Management

Study Questions

- *Which patients with an eating disorder are likely to get the refeeding syndrome?*
- *What will you do if a patient becomes acutely short of breath early in refeeding?*

The physical manifestations of eating disorders (EDs) result from malnutrition, the pathophysiologic consequences of malnutrition, behaviours used to cause weight loss, self-injurious behaviour, and iatrogenic causes. Table 13.1 lists the physical complications of EDs that require specific treatment, and Table 13.2 lists those for which no specific treatment exists. An algorithm for the management of patients with anorexia nervosa (AN) by the primary physician is shown in Figure 13.1. Figure 13.2 shows an algorithm for the treatment of BN by the primary physician.

The Medical Goals of Therapy

- Build rapport, hope for recovery, and faith in treatment.
- Assess and treat coexistent nutritional deficiencies.
- Diagnose comorbid physical conditions (e.g., hyperthyroidism, celiac disease).
- Assess and treat the effects of malnutrition (e.g., osteoporosis).
- Develop healthy eating habits, reduce binge and purge behaviour, gradually reach a healthy weight (total body fat).
- Uncover and treat complications of weight loss behaviours (e.g., erosion of teeth).
- Recognise and treat self-injurious behaviour (e.g., bruising, cutting, self-phlebotomy).
- Prevent, diagnose, and treat complications of treatment (e.g., habituation to anxiolytics).
- Ensure the patient seeks appropriate family therapy, psychological therapy, or psychiatric therapy.

Beginning Treatment

- Build rapport and develop a therapeutic alliance.
- Family involvement and treatment is necessary if the patient's life is family centred.
- Set nutritional goals that begin with small incremental changes from their present eating habits.
- Exercise should be discussed, understood, and limited or changed so it burns fewer calories. When exercise addiction is present, it becomes another comorbid condition that must be treated.

Table 13.1 Medical complications of eating disorders for which there is a specific treatment

Symptom	Cause
Sores at sides of the mouth	Riboflavin deficiency
Bleeding, friable gums	Scurvy
Dry skin, especially on palms of the hands and soles of feet	Zinc deficiency
Nystagmus or ophthalmoplegia	Wernicke's encephalopathy
Confusion or forgetfulness	Drug toxicity; low serum sodium; magnesium, phosphate, vitamin B_{12}, glucose or thiamine deficiency
Symmetrical proximal weakness Seizures	Magnesium, potassium, phosphate, or calcium deficiency
Loss of consciousness or coma	Hypoglycaemia, overdose, Wernicke's encephalopathy, severe hyponatraemia, central pontine myelolysis
Latent tetany with a Chvostek's, Trousseau's or lateral peroneal nerve tap sign	Magnesium deficiency; less likely, potassium deficiency, alkalaemia
Causalgia (an intense burning feeling)	Peripheral neuropathy (alcohol, diabetes mellitus and recovering compression neuropathy are the most common causes of a causalgic neuropathy)
Decreased sensation, peripheral neuropathy	Vitamin B_{12} deficiency, thiamine deficiency, malnutrition, pressure neuropathy
Foot drop	Nerve compression of the lateral peroneal nerve
Mitral valve prolapse murmur	Normally present in 17 per cent of healthy young females, worsens with weight loss, and improves with weight gain If it is associated with the murmur of mitral regurgitation, it can predispose to dysrhythmia and bacterial endocarditis
Dysrhythmias	Low potassium, magnesium, calcium; autonomic dysfunction, QT prolongation, volume depletion, coexistent hyperthyroidism
Postural hypotension	Volume depletion
Pitting oedema	Refeeding syndrome, hypoalbuminaemia
Abdominal tenderness	Obstipation, superior mesenteric artery syndrome, pancreatitis
Bone pain	Fracture, stress fracture, osteomalacia

Table 13.2 Medical complications of eating disorders with no specific treatment

Symptom	Cause/Notes
Generalised alopecia	Severe malnutrition; will reverse with recovery
Aphthous ulcers	No specific cause
Erosion of teeth and gingivitis	Purging
Swelling of sides of face	Can be due to purging and malnutrition independent of purging Stop purging, dehydrate, and can use the sucking of lemons and warming (increased parasympathetic tone)
Lanugo hair	Reverses with weight restoration
Hypercarotenaemia	Due to slow metabolism of carotene Of no pathological consequence Reverses with recovery
Russell's sign	Scarring over the back of the hand due to habitual pressure on the teeth while purging No treatment except stop purging and some dermatologists will inject steroids
Acrocyanosis	Warm and volume replete

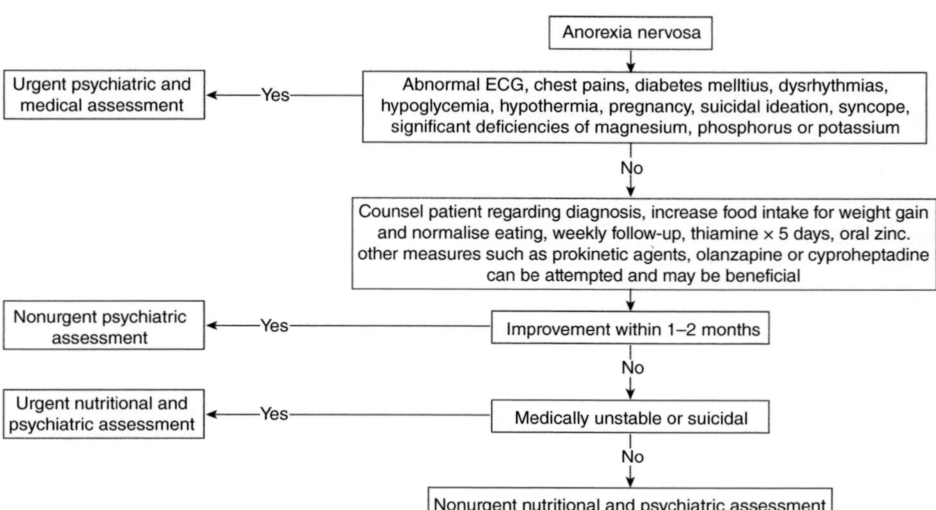

Figure 13.1 Algorithm for the management of anorexia nervosa in primary care. ECG, electrocardiogram.

- Binge and purge behaviour should be monitored and goals for normalisation discussed. However, remember that the initiation of treatment and change in food intake will increase stress, which normally increases the likelihood of binging and purging short term.

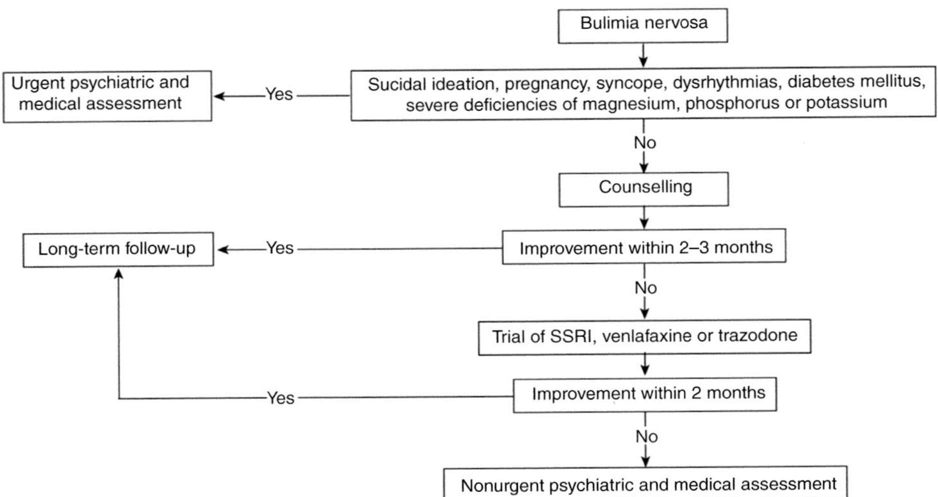

Figure 13.2 Algorithm for the management of bulimia nervosa in primary care.

- Laxative dependency can often be treated using prucalopride 1–2 mg/day during a period of increased water and fibre intake. Prucalopride is a prokinetic agent that causes the large bowel (colon) to contract normally by stimulating the Vagus nerve that innervates the colon. Occasionally, patients will have too marked an effect with abdominal cramps. In that case, prucalopride should be given once a week at a dose of 1 mg and increased in frequency gradually as needed.

Another form of treatment for laxative dependency is vagus nerve stimulation that can be performed by 10 Hz AC stimulation of the left ear by the protocol used to treat migraine headaches or prevent seizures in some patients with epilepsy. Some patients do not want to use prucalopride or vagus nerve stimulation and can be treated with the traditional tapering of laxatives by tapering the laxatives very slowly (over months to years; Table 13.3).

Treat Early

Weight loss, malnutrition, and complications like loss of teeth and osteoporosis can be prevented by early diagnosis and treatment. When rapid weight loss has occurred or when body weight is extremely low, medical instability and death are more likely.

Recurrent vomiting, misuse of laxatives, enemas, suppositories, diuretics, ipecac, self-phlebotomy or gavage, overexercise, ipecac, and underuse of insulin in patients with insulin-dependent diabetes can lead to volume depletion, electrolyte abnormalities, vitamin and mineral deficiencies, and organ dysfunction. Signs and symptoms of medical instability that indicate the need for full medical assessment are listed in Table 13.4.

If medical instability is present, stabilisation is begun using bed rest, intravenous fluids if needed, and correction of deficiencies. Routine administration of a multivitamin, thiamine, phosphorus, potassium, and oral magnesium is mandatory Correction of

Table 13.3 Laxative withdrawal protocol

See Constipation Protocol.
Discontinue all stimulant laxatives.
Begin prucalopride 1 mg/day in the morning. If there is less than adequate effect after a few days increase to 2 mg/day.
Encourage patient to: Increase water intake to 2 l/day. Normalise fibre take to the equivalent of 1–3 tablespoons of crude fibre daily taken with meals.
Use warming protocol. Use warming pad or jacket on medium heat (high setting will have the opposite effect).
Use during meals for 1 hour three times a day.
Supplement diet with prunes or prune delight (three-quarters of a cup of prunes, dates, raisins; one-half cup of orange juice; and one-third cup of water). Simmer on medium low heat until consistency of jam, mix in food processor. Dates to use in prune delight, 20–30 Medjool dates a day.
Ask the patient to resist the temptation to take other laxatives because this will stop the treatment from working. The feelings of bloating, fullness, and constipation are common until normal peristalsis and bowel habit return.
Monitor bowel movements, bowel sounds, and/or flatulence.

Table 13.4 Indications for immediate medical assessment

Indication	Description
Weight loss	Inability to eat or keep down food or rapid weight loss (more than 4 kg over 1 month)
Temperature	Core temperature <35.5°C
Neurological	Confusion, syncope, loss or decreased level of consciousness, organic brain syndrome, ophthalmoplegia, seizure, tetany, ataxia
Cardiac	Palpitations that cause symptoms like light-headedness or chest pain or any ventricular arrhythmia, abnormal pacemaker, QTc of greater than 450 msec, increased heart rate variability (on spectral analysis of electrocardiogram), angina pectoris, heart failure
Metabolic	Renal failure with increasing creatinine or urine output less than 400 ml/day (oliguria), serum sodium <127 mmol/l, potassium <2.3 mmol/l, hypoglycaemia (blood glucose <2.5 mmol/l), hypophosphataemia (phosphorus below normal on fasting sample), magnesium less than 0.6 mmol/l (normal greater than 0.7 mmol/l)
Muscular	Rapidly diminishing exercise tolerance (owing to muscular weakness not accounted for by a correctable deficiency or diaphragmatic wasting)
Pregnancy	The foetus is at risk
Diabetes mellitus	Blood glucose control almost always requires an inpatient admission to control eating behaviour, activity, and insulin without putting the patient at risk for hypoglycaemia

volume (dehydration), electrolytes, and minerals should precede refeeding (see Nutritional Therapy [Refeeding]). Serum potassium, magnesium, and phosphorus should be measured daily for the first week and then three times a week. If the patient is volume depleted normal saline (0.9 per cent sodium chloride) should be given. The rate of intravenous fluids given must be assessed individually.

Do not administer intravenous dextrose until thiamine has been administered, because the intravenous sugar can precipitate acute thiamine deficiency resulting in Wernicke's encephalopathy. Once thiamine has been administered, 5 per cent dextrose in 0.9 per cent saline or 3.3 per cent dextrose in 0.3 per cent saline can be administered, if needed. Serum creatinine, potassium, magnesium, and phosphate should be measured and treated if abnormal.

The administration of glucose is necessary when hypoglycaemia causes seizures, arrhythmia, or loss of consciousness during feeding. Hypoglycaemia occurs when the pancreas releases more insulin in response to the increased carbohydrate intake. This release causes the blood glucose to decrease. Normally, glucose would then be released from the liver by the action of glucagon released from the pancreas. However, if there is insufficient carbohydrate stored in the liver to correct the decrease, hypoglycaemia will occur. Hypoglycaemia is diagnosed when the serum glucose is less than 2.5 mmol/l.

If renal function is impaired or if the patient has not passed urine, potassium should not be administered, or hyperkalaemia may occur. Potassium can be started once the patient begins urinating. Remember, the underweight patient should have a creatinine that is lower than normal – so even a normal creatinine may be a sign of renal insufficiency. Check for renal insufficiency by comparing the creatinine against a previous measurement, if available.

Cardiac chest pain (see Chapter 4) or arrhythmia should prompt immediate investigation. If frequent ventricular premature beats, a prolonged QT interval (greater than 450 msec or an increase of 60 msec beyond baseline electrocardiogram [EKG]) occurs in the setting of marked hypokalaemia, hypomagnesemia, or hypophosphatemia, cardiac monitoring should be started or a cardiologist consulted. Symptoms of arrhythmia include syncope, collapse, and typical or atypical angina. Therefore, cardiac investigation is necessary for those complaints.

A rapid normalisation of heart rate variability increases the likelihood of arrhythmias. The heart rate should increase with exercise or standing up quickly and decreases with rest. An increased heart rate variability means there are greater variations in heart rate observed over time. Patients with increased heart rate variability may notice that their heart rate goes too slow when they are resting or suddenly goes fast for no reason. They may also notice other symptoms of autonomic dysfunction like intermittent dry mouth, perspiration, and the sudden need to urinate or defecate.

A sudden decrease in heart rate variability predisposes to arrhythmia and sudden death in many medical settings. This usually occurs during refeeding and the patient most often complains of the recent onset of perspiration at a time that they did not perspire before. This symptom should be taken as a symptom of cardiac instability owing to the rapidly changing effect of the stress response from the brain.

The calorie content of feeding that starts after the stabilisation process must begin slowly and be monitored carefully. The fewer the calories to start and the more slowly the calories are increased the safer.

Hospital Treatment for the Medically Unstable Patient

- Bed rest
- Intravenous fluids and minerals as necessary
- Correction of deficiencies
- Refeeding after deficiencies are corrected and dehydration is corrected
- Begin refeeding slowly to avoid the refeeding syndrome (unmasking latent deficiencies with a load of macronutrients (carbohydrates, fats, proteins)
- Methods of feeding: meal support is preferred with meals prescribed by a dietician working with the patient. Meals are usually begun at about 1200 calories a day. ft the patient is severely malnourished begin at 600 kcal/day. If the patient is unable to eat, use supplements, behavioural strategies, or nasogastric feeding. Occasionally, gastrostomy feedings are the only route acceptable to the patient. The fact the tube is bypassing the mouth seems to make it more acceptable.
- During refeeding aimed at weight gain: supplements of thiamine 100 mg for 5 days, multivitamins daily, KCL 20 mEq twice a day, phosphorus 500 mg twice a day, and zinc citrate 50 mg of elemental zinc daily, monitor potassium, phosphorus, and magnesium daily for 5–7 days and then three times a week unless levels are dropping, then continue daily measurements (Table 13.5).

Caution

- Hypoglycaemia can occur during refeeding because insulin secretion is stimulated by food intake when there is still inadequate liver glycogen to be released by glucagon to prevent the low blood sugar.
- Hypophosphatemia can occur rapidly. If the phosphate level drops, the amount of oral phosphate should be increased stepwise and the level measured at least once daily. If the level continues to decrease, discontinue all feeding and give oral and intravenous phosphate.
- Hyponatremia: a serum sodium lower than 125 mmol/l must be corrected slowly. Rapid correction of hyponatremia, particularly in malnourished patients, can cause cerebral oedema resulting in a decreased level of consciousness and occasionally death of part of the brain stem (central pontine myelolysis). Central pontine myelolysis is often fatal.

Medications

- Prokinetic medications: domperidone or metoclopramide help to reduce early satiety, abdominal discomfort, and oesophageal reflux. Domperidone and metoclopramide have equivalent dosages, begin with 5 mg and gradually increase to 20 mg if required to relieve symptoms. The medication should be given 15–30 minutes before meals because that is how long it takes them to act. Both drugs can cause the extrapyramidal side effects of the other major tranquilisers. However, only a small amount of domperidone crosses the blood–brain barrier, so it is much less likely to cause side effects. Therefore, use domperidone unless the patient has nausea; nausea is decreased by metoclopramide but not domperidone. Both drugs can cause galactorrhoea (breast milk) by increasing prolactin release from the pituitary. This side effect is not dangerous, but the patient may wish to stop the medication because of the galactorrhoea or the increase in breast size.

Table 13.5 Medical admission orders for the patient with an eating disorder

Encourage rest (specify limitations to activity, e.g., wheelchair only, no physical activity, no passes off the ward)
Dietitian to order diet
Admission laboratory work: Haemoglobin, white blood cell count, platelets, serum sodium, potassium, chloride, bicarbonate, blood urea nitrogen, creatinine, CPK, aspartate transaminase, alkaline phosphatase, magnesium, calcium, phosphorus, ferritin, vitamin B_{12}, red blood cell folate, zinc, International Normalised Ratio (INR)
Electrocardiogram
Urinalysis (midstream urine)
Hypnotic as required: zoplicone 7.5–15.0 mg at bedtime or chloral hydrate 500 mg to 1000 mg at bedtime, or trazodone 12.5–50 mg at bedtime or clonazepam 0.5–2.0 mg at bedtime
Be aware of the amnestic and disinhibiting effects of benzodiazepines
Anxiolytics: Lorazepam 0.5–2.0 mg sublingually up to every hour as required or clonazepam 0.5–2.0 mg orally up to 4 times a day or quetiapine 25–50 mg every 6 hours as required; quetiapine has extrapyramidal side effects
Repeat blood work: potassium, phosphorus, and magnesium daily for 7 days and then every Monday, Wednesday, and Friday
Daily blood work should be continued or restarted if a deficiency occurs in any of these three minerals
Standard supplements
Potassium chloride (pills, effervescent, or liquid) 24 mEq three times a day for 21 days
Sodium phosphate solution 5 ml (550 mg of phosphorus) three times a day for 21 days; continue once a day if weight gain continues at a rate of more than 0.5 kg a week
Multivitamin 2 tablets a day for 2 months and then 1 tablet a day
Thiamine 100 mg/day for 5 days; thiamine 100 mg intramuscular or intravenous must be given if glucose is to be given intravenously
Zinc gluconate approximately 100 mg/day (contains 14 mg of elemental zinc) for 2 months
Intravenous rehydration: if dehydrated, give normal saline (0.9 per cent NaCl solution) at 100–150 ml/hour until intravascular volume is normalised based on jugular venous pressure and postural change in heart rate and blood pressure
Bowel routine: Fibre such as crude bran 3–7 tablespoons a day; at least 2 litres a day of fluid intake
If the patient has abused laxatives consider prucalopride 1 mg/day (see Bowel Protocols)
Domperidone or metoclopramide 5 to10 mg one-half hour before meals (three times a day) and at bedtime and titrate dose upward in 5-mg increments
Use domperidone in preference to metoclopramide, which is more likely to cause extrapyramidal side effects

- Prokinetic agents of the large bowel (colon): Prucalopride is a prokinetic agent that stimulates the parasympathic nerves that cause the large bowel to contract. Like domperidone and meclopromide, which effect the oesophagus, stomach, and duodenum, the mechanism of action of prucalopride strengthens the large bowel. This is similar to the way that exercise strengthens the muscles. Prucalopride has largely replaced the need for laxative taper. It is immediately effective from the first use. Because the medication strengthens the bowel, it should be used for 1–3 months before attempting to taper it. Patients who have used laxatives for decades may require the medication for years. The dosage is 1 or 2 mg once a day. Decrease the dose if the 2-mg dose causes cramps. Prucalopride should not be used if there is a bowel obstruction or partial obstruction.
- Medications for obstipation: When the patient has a partial obstruction of their large bowel due to hard stool in their rectum or entire colon, a series of medications and procedures are necessary. Even in hospital, this phase of treatment may take weeks to a few months. Occasionally and wrongly, a colectomy is performed instead.
  1. Correct dehydration by giving fluids. Normalise deficiencies including electrolytes. Measure and correct magnesium and calcium. If the patient is taking iron, this should be held because it may worsen the constipation.
  2. A digital rectal examination should be performed by a medical doctor to check for rectal prolapse and the consistency of the stool. Usually there is little or no rectal prolapse but there are small hard stools.
  3. Use enemas to clear the lower bowel. If an enema is effective, continue it using it once or twice a day until it is no longer needed or try the next type of enema. The oil retention enema can always be used before any other enema if it can be held for 30 minutes to lubricate the bowel. Enemas in suggested order or use are:

     a. Saline enema,
     b. Oil retention enema,
     c. Dulcolax Microenema, and
     d. Soap suds enema with 30 ml of Castile soap in 1,000–1,500 ml of water.

  4. Bulk forming agents: Bulk-forming agents bind water to give bulk and thereby help normalise bowel function. They should be taken regularly to be effective. Dioctylsodiumsulfasuccinate, Metamucil, or similar agents are prescribed daily in conjunction with a fluid intake of at least 2 l/day.

- Prune juice or 'prune delight' to maintain regular bowel movements during the change in the intake try

  - Prune Delight recipe: Three-quarters of a cup of prunes, dates, and raisins; one-half of a cup of orange juice; one-third of a cup of water. Simmer on medium low heat until consistency of jam and mix in a food processor. Dates in prune delight are 20–30 Medjool dates.

- Anxiolytics: Benzodiazepines are usually avoided. Most psychiatrists prefer antipsychotics for the treatment of sleep and anxiety. When benzodiazepines are used owing to choice or side effects of antipsychotics, the most commonly used in benzodiazepines are lorazepam and clonazepam. Lorazepam can be used to treat acute anxiety and clonazepam can be used to treat constant anxiety. However, benzodiazepines are habituating, can cause amnesia, and can cause emotional lability. Clonazepam is usually begun at 0.5 mg twice a day and titrated upward every few days as required. The maximum dose of clonazepam is 20 mg/day. However, habituation is more likely with higher dosages and longer medication use, particularly in outpatients.

- Quetiapine is a major tranquiliser that is effective in reducing anxiety in AN. It is not habituating, does not cause amnesia, and does not cause emotional lability. However, it is sedating and has all the potential side effects of other major tranquilisers, including extrapyramidal side effects. Quetiapine is usually started at 25 mg twice a day with the dosage increased gradually.
- Antidepressants: There is little evidence that antidepressants are effective for mood or weight gain in low weight AN. The major indication for antidepressants is the treatment of a coexistent major depression once weight restoration has progressed. They can also be used in an attempt to lessen bingeing and purging behaviour. Serotonin reuptake inhibitors are the preferred antidepressants in EDs because they are effective and have less toxicity than tricyclic antidepressants and monoaminoxidase inhibitors. Serotonin reuptake inhibitors can be used to treat major depression, binge-purge behaviour, and coexistent obsessive–compulsive disorder. Do not use tricyclic antidepressants or monoaminoxidase inhibitors because of their toxicity. Bupropion is relatively contraindicated because it increases the risk of seizures in patients with and ED. This is mostly in those who binge and purge. If patients who have binge–purge behaviour purge after taking the medication, they may take a second dose and this makes toxicity much more likely.
- Cyproheptadine can increase weight gain. The only patients who are willing to take it are those with chronic AN who want to increase their quality of life but refuse admission or use of olanzapine. Cyproheptadine should be taken at bedtime, because it is sedating. Start with a dose of 4 mg and increase, if tolerated, to 16 mg.
- Major tranquilisers – olanzapine, quetiapine, risperidone, and loxapine – can be used in the treatment of AN. Of these, only olanzapine routinely causes a marked reduction in the ruminative thinking of AN. Often olanzapine is effective at very low dosages of 2.5–7.5 mg. When any major tranquiliser is used, monitor the extrapyramidal side effects and adjust the dose downward or discontinue if they occur.
- Zinc: Zinc supplementation increases the rate of weight gain irrespective of the serum zinc level. Oral zinc should be given in a dose of 50 mg of elemental zinc a day as zinc citrate. There is insufficient zinc in multivitamins. Zinc causes gastric upset in about 2 per cent of patients; this is reduced by taking the pills with meals. Serum zinc does not reflect brain zinc; there is no brain store of zinc and the daily intake of zinc effects brain function such as food seeking. The main food source of zinc is cow's milk and seafood.
- Ondansetron has not been shown to be useful in preventing purging.

Notes

- Normal body fat is usually necessary for psychological or medication therapy to be effective.
- The response of individual patients to antidepressants is highly variable. Lack of success or side effects with one antidepressant does not mean other antidepressants

Table 13.6 Risks associated with medications

Medication	Associated Risks
Marijuana	Commonly used for recreational and therapeutic reasons. It is taken in many forms that have different effects and side effects. There are many subtypes of cannabinoid receptors in the brain and the metabolism is slow. Psychosis, paranoia, panic, and bizarre behaviour may follow the use or discontinuance of marijuana or its products.
Bupropion	Can cause seizures in eating disorders.
Serotonin reuptake inhibitors	Can lead to the serotonergic syndrome if used to excess doses, combined or if the metabolism is reduced through drug interactions.
Major tranquilisers including quetiapine, olanzapine, metoclopramide, domperidone, and antinausea medications like trilafon.	Can cause extrapyramidal side effects like Parkinsonism, akathisia, tardive dyskinesia, malignant neuroleptic syndrome, and galactorrhoea.
Herbal remedies	May have the action of laxatives, diuretics, steroids, and other active agents.
Stimulants (like ephedrine, they may be used covertly to promote weight loss)	Can lower the threshold to seizures and arrhythmias. Withdrawal symptoms occur if stopped suddenly.
Benzodiazepines	To avoid withdrawal, including seizures, taper no faster than 20 per cent a day.
Alcohol	Be aware of alcohol withdrawal.
Habituation	Be aware of addiction in patients with a history of addiction.
Overdose	Many patients with anorexia nervosa stockpile medications or have access to medications of others. Monitor medication use, multidoctoring and drug hoarding.

will not be effective. South East Asian patients may genetically not metabolise some antidepressants – leading to high blood levels and toxicity. Very low dosages (e.g., 1–5 mg of fluoxetine a day) may be necessary. If family members of your patient have been successfully treated with specific antidepressants, it is more likely to be effective in them.

- In AN the total body fat mass is low, the lean body mass is more nearly normal, the renal and liver function are usually normal, and the metabolic rate is often high. The volume of distribution of drugs and the dose of drugs required is often as high as, or higher than, normal weight patients.
- Before ordering a drug, consider its effect on cardiac function. Drugs that prolong the QT interval should be avoided or the ECG should be reassessed during their use.
- Risks associated with medications used in EDs are listed in Table 13.6

Laboratory Investigations

Laboratory investigations that should be ordered include a complete blood count, electrolytes, blood urea nitrogen, creatinine, magnesium, phosphorus, calcium, creatine phosphokinase, AST, alkaline phosphatase, ferritin, red blood cell folate, vitamin B_{12}, thyroid-stimulating hormone, EKG, and urinalysis.

Laboratory Investigations That Should Be Repeated

EKG

Repeat the EKG weekly, but daily if the QTc is longer than 460 msec. Magnesium, phosphorus, potassium daily should be repeated for 5–7 days and then every Monday, Wednesday, and Friday for 21 days (or until the patient stops gaining weight).

Blood Glucose

Test the blood glucose when the patient is admitted for AN, if they have symptoms consistent with hypoglycaemia after meals, or if they have sweating, nightmares, or confusion during the night. Do a chemstrip as soon as you suspect hypoglycaemia and do glucose testing with chemstrips between 30 minutes and 1.5 hours after eating when diet is increased or with symptoms of hypoglycaemia or a change in mentation or behaviour after meals. Hypoglycaemia is defined clinically as a serum glucose of less than 2.5 mmol/L, or a chemstrip of less than 2.5 mmol/l associated with symptoms of hypoglycemia (e.g., confusion, lightheadedness, decreased coordination, or failing a glucagon test). Once diagnosed with hypoglycaemia, and until the glucagon test is passed, blood glucose should continue to be measured by chemstrip 30 minutes to 1.5 hours after meals.

When Should a Glucagon Test Be Performed?

1. You suspect hypoglycaemia but lack the resources to document it.
2. You want to exclude hypoglycaemia as the cause of unexplained seizures, loss of consciousness, or arrhythmias.
3. You want to stop special treatment (dietary, nasogastric tube, or intravenous) for hypoglycaemia, but you must ensure the patient has recovered their liver glycogen first.

Glucagon Test

a. Preparation: Have intravenous access available; fast for at least 3–4 hours before testing in the morning.
b. Measure blood glucose before, 10 minutes, and 20 minutes after glucagon injection.
c. Inject glucagon 1 mg intravenously as a push and then flush with 10 ml normal saline.
d. Interpretation: A normal test: the blood glucose increases from the baseline on either subsequent reading to either greater than 6.5mmol/l with a 2 mmol/l increase or greater than 7mmol/l.

Important Reminders

- The intravenous access line must be flushed with normal saline, not dextrose.
- The glucagon must be completely dissolved before administering.

- The intravenous access must be completely flushed with saline before and after administration of the glucagon.

Laboratory blood glucose measurement is very accurate at all levels of glucose. Needle prick measurement is not accurate when the blood glucose is less than 3 mmol/l and at low levels may have an error as large as 2 mmol/l. Therefore, needle prick glucose measurement should only be used as a screening test for hypoglycaemia, not for the glucagon test.

Nutritional Therapy (Refeeding)

- The dietitian should assess and begin feeding at a rate of 600–1200 kcal/day. Gradually increase according to previous caloric requirements for refeeding, or every few days until the caloric content is at least 1,800–2,200 kcal a day or more as required to achieve a weight gain of 1 kg a week (approximately 1 per cent body fat gain a week).
- Refeeding for a patient with hypoglycaemia: Continuous enteral feeding should be used until the glucagon test is passed.
- If hypoglycaemia is diagnosed, there is a continuing risk of hypoglycaemia during refeeding. Continuous enteral feeding must be used to prevent hypoglycaemia, until the patient has a normal glucagon test.
- Tube feeding is more reliable and successful at preventing hypoglycaemia than regular diet or intravenous feeding. The rate of feeding will vary depending on the rate required to prevent hypoglycaemia, the ability of the patient to eat, and the number of calories required for weight gain.
- If tube feeding is interrupted in a patient being treated for hypoglycaemia: Start an intravenous infusion of 10 per cent dextrose in water at 100 ml per hour. The rate should be titrated to prevent hypoglycaemia.
- Give thiamine (vitamin B_1) 100 mg immediately and 100 mg/day for 5 days.

Potassium

Give 20 mmol of potassium chloride three times a day by mouth, during refeeding. Correct the causes of potassium loss, which include dehydration, magnesium deficiency, and potassium wasting diuretics.

a. Normal potassium, normal creatinine, gaining weight: 20 mEq two to three times a day of oral potassium.
b. Potassium decreasing but within normal limits, normal creatinine, gaining weight: Increase the dose of potassium orally and recheck in 1–2 days.
c. Potassium below normal, normal creatinine, gaining weight: Start as in (a) and titrate upward. If the potassium does not increase, change to intravenous potassium at 40 mmol/l of KCl in 1000 ml or 0.9 per cent saline at 150 cc/hr and titrate to serum potassium.
d. Potassium less than 2.2 mmol/l with possible symptoms of potassium deficiency (palpitations, muscle weakness), EKG abnormalities consistent with potassium deficiency (e.g., T wave height diminishing): Refer to medicine, collect urine for potassium concentration, have intravenous access ready.

Do Not Administer Potassium until the Patient Has Voided

If the serum potassium continues to decrease or stays low despite potassium supplementation, check urine potassium (should be very low, i.e., less than 5mmol/l; if it is higher, correct volume depletion with normal saline intravenously and totally body magnesium depletion with magnesium infusions).

Magnesium

Magnesium repletion can be achieved with black strap molasses. Previously magnesium was given intravenously because all of the oral routes were inadequately absorbed. However, it is clear that black strap molasses can be used to treat and prevent magnesium deficiency – except for magnesium deficiency in the setting of seizure, arrhythmia, Wernicke's encephalopathy, or other life-endangering situation. In those situations, intravenous magnesium should still be used as outlined.

The initial crush of sugar cane yields black strap molasses that has a great deal of magnesium and iron as well as other nutrients. Three tablespoons a day (15 ml = 1 tablespoon) is adequate to treat and prevent magnesium deficiency. One tablespoon contains about 90 kcal and it does taste sweet, so some patients will refuse to take it. Because of its sweetness it is best ingested with tea, applesauce, or any other food that the patient likes the taste of. It delivers the magnesium whether taken by itself, in drinks, or used in cooking.

The intravenous infusions of 20 mm of magnesium sulphate in 250 ml of normal saline is accomplished over 3–4 hours daily for 5–7 days. To see whether more infusions are needed do a balance or load test with the last infusion. Low serum magnesium always means there is a significant total body deficiency of magnesium. In addition, total body deficiency is often present with normal serum magnesium. A magnesium load test should be performed to diagnose total body magnesium deficiency if there are symptoms of muscle cramps, muscle weakness, loss of visual accommodation after reading for half an hour, or impaired short-term memory. The routes of administration and dosage of magnesium are shown in Table 13.7.

Magnesium Load (or Balance) Test

a. Have the patient completely empty their bladder. Then begin a 24-hour urine collection for total magnesium and creatinine content.
b. Administer an intravenous infusion of 20 mmol of magnesium sulphate in 250 ml of normal saline (or 500–1000 ml if they are dehydrated).
c. Decide whether the urine was collected for 24 hours, as was the plan. The urine volume should be 700–1000 ml unless the patient is dehydrated, and the total urine creatinine which should be about 5–7 mmol/day in AN. If the urine creatinine is too low, the urine collection is incomplete; if the urine creatinine is much higher, urine was collected for too long. Either way – start over.
d. If there is 18 mol or more of magnesium in the collection, there is no deficiency present and no further infusions are needed (rarely this result is due to kidney dysfunction causing an inability to reabsorb magnesium, irrespective of total body magnesium). If there is less than 16 mmol of magnesium in the urine collection, the patient is still deficient. A urine collection with 16–18 mmol is indeterminate.
    - Proton pump inhibitors: medications that reduce stomach acid like omeprazole, pantoprazole, lansoprazole, and esomeprazole inhibit magnesium absorption in the bowel in a small percentage of patients. Many patients with chronic EDs take

Table 13.7 Magnesium supplementation

Route	Medications	Orders	Benefits and Limitations
Oral	Magnesium Black strap molasses	Fifteen millilitres three times a day for weeks to months	Black strap molasses is very well-absorbed and has replaced the need for other routes of magnesium supplementation except in emergencies where parenteral magnesium must be used.
Intramuscular	A 10-ml vial of magnesium sulphate 50 per cent solution contains 20 mmol of magnesium, 40 mEq of magnesium, and 5 g of magnesium sulphate	2 ml intramuscularly in one or both buttocks For the treatment of a symptomatic deficiency give one injection hourly for 6 hours and then one injection every 4 hours for 5 days	Fast and inexpensive, the amount incorporated into cells is more than with intravenous because it is absorbed from the intramuscular route more slowly. However, the injections often cause pain and because only; 2 ml can be given intramuscularly, and many injections are required.
Intravenous	Same as intramuscular solution	20 mmol of magnesium sulphate in 250 ml of 09 per cent saline over 4 hours daily for 5–10 days	Increases the serum and tissue levels quickly, resulting in symptomatic improvement. However, the need for daily intravenous infusions limits the availability of treatment. Note: overdosing and underdosing are common because: 40 mEq of magnesium = 20mmol of magnesium = 10 ml of 50 per cent solution = 5 g of magnesium sulphate

these medications. If your patient has a magnesium deficiency these medications should be stopped. Diuretics cause magnesium loss in the urine, except for amiloride, eplerenone, spironolactone, and triamterene. If your patient has magnesium deficiency and is on a diuretic, consider changing the diuretic.

Phosphorus

Phosphate is absorbed rapidly and easily from the bowel. The serum level of phosphate increases briefly after a meal containing phosphate and then falls. Thus, serum phosphate should be measured fasting. If serum phosphate is slightly low as measured in an outpatient ask, whether the blood was drawn after a meal.

Phosphate is part of ATP, the primary source of energy for all of the cells in our body. A patient with a slightly low phosphate will have no symptoms. When phosphate falls to between one-half and one-third of the lower limit of normal, it is like the power cord is pulled on the vacuum. Heart failure occurs – along with failure of most organ systems (e.g., rhabdomyolysis, haemolytic anaemia), followed by death. Thus, prevention is necessary for hypophosphatemia – treatment of severe hypophosphatemia is too late. A litre of skim milk has 500 mg of phosphate.

Prevention of Hypophosphatemia

1. During refeeding if the serum phosphate is normal and stable, give phosphate 500 mg three times a day as liquid or tablet.
2. During refeeding if the serum phosphate is normal but decreasing, give a stepwise increase in oral phosphate (e.g., to 1000 mg four times a day) and measure serum phosphate daily.
3. During refeeding if the serum phosphate is slightly low (more than 70 per cent of normal) but steady, increase the dose of oral phosphate and measure phosphate twice daily. In addition, measure the concentration of phosphate in the urine to make sure it is not being wasted (about 20 per cent of patients waste phosphate in the urine if they are hypomagnesemia – so you would have to treat the magnesium as well).
4. If the serum phosphate is low (less than 70 per cent of normal) and falling, but there are no symptoms, stop feeding until the serum phosphate is normal, change intravenous fluid to normal saline (intravenous dextrose will lower serum phosphate), give 1000 mg phosphate orally four times a day, give intravenous phosphate, and consult the intensive care unit.
5. If the serum phosphate is low and there are associated symptoms (e.g., shortness of breath, weakness, seizure, marked fatigue) as in (4) and transfer to the intensive care unit.

Warming Protocols

Most patients who take holidays in very warm places report feeling better during the vacation. Research shows that warming helps to improve bowel function, reduce anxiety, reduce parotid size, and reduce activity. Warming also normalises autonomic dysfunction. Warming reduces non-exercise activity thermogenesis! Patients who have these micromovements (standing all the time, standing and sitting, bouncing their legs, tensing their muscles) may be expending another 2000 kcal/day. If you use warming or put them in a 40°C room, the micromovements will decrease or disappear – resulting in weight gain!

Warming Jacket or Warming Pad Protocol

1. Warming jacket setting: Medium.
2. When: Preferably during meals (can be used at other times in addition but not during sleep).
3. Duration: 1 hour, 3 times a day.

Sauna Protocol for Inpatients

1. Measure blood pressure. (Patients with a systolic blood pressure of less than 85 mm Hg should not enter the sauna).
2. The patient should then change into a hospital gown. Set the temperature on the sauna to start at 30°C (86°F) and to stop at 45°C (113°F).

3. The patient should consume one glass of water before entering the sauna.
4. Allow the patient to remain in the sauna for a maximum of 10 minutes. They may leave the door open a crack to allow for air circulation.
5. Measure blood pressure on exiting the sauna.
6. The patient should take a shower, during which they should gradually decrease the water temperature to room temperature. They are not to take a cold shower.

Sauna Protocol for Outpatients

1. No alcohol consumption.
2. Blood pressure must be taken and recorded before and after the sauna (persons with blood pressure below 85 mm Hg systolic symptomatic hypotension, or postural hypotension should not use the sauna).
3. One glass of water must be consumed before entering the sauna.
4. The patient should then change into a bathing suit or gown. Set the temperature on the sauna to start at 30°C (86°F) and to stop at 45°C (113°F). Allow the patient to stay in the sauna for a maximum of 10 minutes.
5. Upon exiting the sauna, measure blood pressure again.
6. No cold showers after the sauna.
7. Sauna may be used from once a week to daily.

Parotid Protocol

The parotid protocol is used to help decrease the size of enlarged parotid glands. Use a warming jacket or sauna protocol plus rinse the mouth thoroughly after each meal. Using a lemon-flavoured liquid can speed the process by increasing the flow of saliva. Do not use lemon if it causes soreness of the teeth.

Fluids

Intravenous Fluid Repletion

Treatment included normal saline 0.9 per cent sodium chloride, initial bolus of 250–500 cc then 150 ml/hour until the dehydration is corrected. Intravenous dextrose can precipitate Wernicke's encephalopathy if thiamine, magnesium or phosphate are deficient. Give thiamine 100 mg intramuscularly and intravenously before starting an intravenous dextrose infusion. Dehydrated patients have a low jugular venous pressure and/or a postural drop in blood pressure or increase in heart rate). Psychotropic medications may cause that same change in blood pressure and heart rate dehydration.

Oral Fluid Repletion

Dehydration with dizziness on standing, a blood pressure drop on standing, or decreased urine output can be treated in reliable patients as an outpatient if the symptoms are still mild. Treatment is three cups a day of high salt (about 50 mEq NaCl) oxo or bouillon or miso in addition to 3 litres of fluid a day. This is equivalent of one litre of normal saline that contains about 154 mEq per litre. The salt remains in the blood. That is why it is essential and why drinking water, which dilutes out to 60 per cent of the body does not work by itself.

Fullness

Fullness or early satiety means that the patient feels full after eating even a little food. It is usually caused by less than normal activity of the stomach and bowel, which is caused by malnutrition or vomiting. Occasionally, it is due to decreased intestinal peristalsis due to deficiency of potassium, magnesium, calcium, constipation, or hypothyroidism. Rarely, if it is severe it may be due to superior mesenteric artery syndrome.

Treatment

1. Warming jacket protocol.
2. Bowel protocol.
3. Prokinetic drugs: domperidone 5–20 mg one-half hour before meals three times a day and at bedtime. If nausea is also present, give meclopramide 5–20 mg one-half hour before meals three times a day and at bedtime instead of domperidone. Erythromycin also has prokinetic effect when given at dose of 125 mg twice a day. Erythromycin can cause nausea and prolong the QT interval. It can be used in addition to domperidone or meclopramide.

Domperidone and meclopramide are both major tranquilisers and can therefore cause hyperprolactinemia, which can result in galactorrhoea and extrapyramidal side effects. Domperidone is preferred because it has fewer extrapyramidal side effects because it crosses the blood–brain barrier much less than meclopramide.

Bloating owing to obstipation in the large bowel can be treated with prucalopride 1–2 mg/day. The prucalopride is a prokinetic agent that causes the large bowel (colon) to contract normally by stimulating the vagus nerve terminals on the colon. Occasionally, patients will have too marked an effect with abdominal cramps, in which case prucalopride should be given once a week at a dose of 1 mg and increased in frequency as needed.

Vagus nerve stimulation can increase intestinal motility. It is performed by stimulating the vagus nerve using 10 Hz AC stimulation of the left ear.

Oedema

1. Moderate oedema is common during the first few weeks of refeeding and mild oedema is common intermittently during the course of disease. This is normal and the patient should be reassured that treatment will cause the oedema to last longer. This is because the body will sense the medications used to treat the oedema as dehydration and will respond with increased fluid retention over a longer period of time.
2. Below knee antiembolic stockings can be used for leg oedema. These must be taken off at night and then put in the morning before rising. If they are not put on in the evening, they will cause stasis of blood and can predispose to blood clots.
3. A low serum albumen causes oedema. If the serum albumen is below normal, the oedema will persist until albumen normalises. Use this information to motivate the patient, telling them that weight gain will normalise the albumen. Low serum albumen is rare in patients with and ED. If the serum albumen is low, check for excess urine loss of albumen and liver dysfunction.

4. If you choose to use a diuretic, spironolactone is the diuretic of choice. Spironolactone does not cause the loss of potassium and magnesium like most other diuretics. It has a gradual onset and offset of action and it is a physiologic aldosterone antagonist, which means it will not work if it is not needed physiologically. The dosage of spironolactone is 50–100 mg/day as a single daily dose.

Criteria for Hospital Treatment before Treatment at a Residential or Outpatient Facility

- Medical or psychiatric condition routinely requiring hospitalisation: such as acute pancreatitis, angina pectoris, heart failure, pneumonia, acute abdomen, or decreasing level of consciousness, psychosis, or acute mania.
- Acute risk of suicide.
- Continued weight loss: Loss of more than 4 kg body weight during the last 2 months.
- Very low body fat: Total body fat less than 10 per cent and not medically stable.
  - Heart: heart failure, second- or third-degree heart block, frequent premature ventricular beats, or arrhythmias causing dizziness or collapse.
- Fasting serum phosphate less than two-thirds of the lower limit of normal.
- Serum potassium of less than 2.5 mmol/L.
- Serum magnesium of less than 0.6 mmol/L.
- Serum sodium of less than 127 mmol/L.
- Serum creatinine greater than the upper limit of normal (usually 110 mmol/l).
- Hypoglycaemia (serum glucose of less than 2.5 mmol/L).
- Core temperature less than 35.5°C.
- Recent seizure unless judged to be stable by a neurologist.
- Recent loss of consciousness or seizure, unless cleared by internist or neurologist.

The presence of any one or more criteria excludes admission to a residential facility or outpatient program until assessed and treated,

These criteria refer to a current condition unless otherwise stated.

Section 6 Treatment

Chapter 14

Managing Medical Complications

Oedema

Case

A 25-year-old woman gains 8 kg in 7 days. She is extremely anxious and agitated, and threatens to discharge herself against medical advice. The nurse asks you why she has gained so much weight.

Comment

During feeding, oedema occurs owing to volume depletion, low metabolic rate, and behaviours such as vomiting, laxative, enema, or diuretic use, which cause the body to have high circulating hormones that promote the retention of fluid. Antidiuretic hormone is secreted by the pituitary, renin by the kidney, angiotensin is formed in the blood, and aldosterone is produced by the adrenal gland. The amount of fluid that will be retained in a patient is impossible to predict, but it is often 3–5 kg. The fluid retention is much greater in those with a history of binge–purge behaviour or diuretic use.

If the patient is suspected of having oedema, apply steady, firm pressure with the pad of your thumb over the skin covering the lower tibia, just about the ankle. After 15 seconds, a small pit will appear if oedema is present. The depth of the pit is roughly proportional to the amount of oedema if the patient has been ambulatory for several hours. If the patient has been lying down, then the oedema will shift to the most dependent area; this is usually the lower back. In this case, apply pressure in the midline over the lumbosacral spine. Occasionally, the patient will lie on their abdomen face down with their arm over the side of the bed. In this case the oedema will be most prominent in the hand and face. Less commonly, oedema is due to hypoalbuminemia (low oncotic pressure, renal failure (high creatinine with associated fluid retention), or heart failure.

Prevention

Normalise the fluid volume on admission. If an intravenous line is not available, then salt-containing cubes dissolved in water can be ingested. As soon as the jugular venous pressure is normalised, discontinue the salt administration. Normally, the process takes 3 days. Rest should be encouraged because recumbency allows the body to clear excess fluid by increasing the glomerular filtration rate. If the risk of oedema is considered high or treatment resistance is felt to be very likely if oedema occurs, give spironolactone 200 mg once a day for 14–21 days. Spironolactone is a weak diuretic that is a physiologic aldosterone antagonist. It often interrupts oedema formation. It also causes potassium and magnesium retention, whereas most other diuretics increase their loss.

Treatment

If oedema develops, reassure the patient that it is temporary and encourage bed rest. Treatment with diuretics often causes cyclic oedema (ongoing recurrent oedema) that may last for a year or more after discontinuing diuretics. If treatment is to be given, treat with spironolactone as described. If the oedema is refractory to spironolactone, then the second-line treatment is an angiotensin-converting enzyme inhibitor. These medications decrease angiotensin formation and thereby aldosterone production.

- Examine for oedema: Press softly with your thumb over a bony prominence of a dependent area to test for pitting oedema.
- Consider refeeding, hypoalbuminemia, congestive heart failure, and renal failure as possible causes.
- Give information and reassurance.
- Encourage bed rest.
- If the oedema leads to treatment resistance or refusal:
  - Give spironolactone 200 mg a day temporarily.
  - Do not give any other diuretic, because they will cause recurrent oedema and thereby diuretic dependency.

Implications for Health Care Professionals

- Reassure the patient that oedema is common and that it usually resolves in 1–2 weeks with no treatment
- Have the patient rest in bed. This measure decreases the oedema by increasing the movement of the oedema fluid into the blood and then excreted as urine.
  - If spironolactone is used, tell the patient it is a diuretic that blocks the cause of the oedema. They will not need it more for than 2–4 weeks.

Aches and Pains

Case

A 28-year-old woman with chronic anorexia nervosa (AN) is seen for aches and pains. She has been stable for several years. A few months ago, she began eating more in an attempt to improve her strength. She began having aches and pains about a month ago. She comes to see you to ask whether you can help.

Comment

'Aches and pains' can mean many different things. You must decide what it means in this patient. It may mean weakness, muscle cramps, numbness, causalgia (burning pain), bone pain, or nonspecific systemic symptoms. Therefore, first ask further questions to define specifically what the problem is. See Table 14.1 for the differential diagnosis.

Table 14.1 Aches and pains

Problem	Syndrome	Causes	Investigations	Treatment
Weakness	Proximal myopathy	Potassium low	Measure serum levels	Treat deficiency
		Phosphorus low	May need to do magnesium load test	
		Magnesium low		
	Neuropathy	Vitamin B_{12} low	Measure serum levels	Treat deficiency and malnutrition; if the cause is pressure neuropathy, consult a neurologist
		Pyridoxine low	Nerve conduction study	
		Malnutrition		
		Pressure neuropathy		
Muscle cramps	Latent tetany	Magnesium low	Measure serum levels	Treat deficiency
	Trousseau's sign, Chvostek's sign, lateral peroneal nerve tap sign	Calcium low	May need to do magnesium load test	
Numbness	Neuropathy	Malnutrition	Physical examination	Treat the specific cause
		Deficiency of vitamin B_{12}, pyridoxine	Nerve conduction study	
		Compression neuropathy		
Causalgia (burning pain)	Neuropathy	Compression, alcohol, or diabetes	Physical examination	Pain can be treated with amitriptyline, dilantin, or Tegretol
			Nerve conduction study	

Table 14.1 *(cont.)*

Problem	Syndrome	Causes	Investigations	Treatment
Bone pains	Osteomalacia	Osteoporosis, osteomalacia are not caused by AN, unless there is a concomitant cause of osteomalacia owing to malnutrition This is usually due to magnesium deficiency	Bone density	Stress fractures should be treated with rest and investigation of the osteoporosis or osteomalacia. Refer to an endocrinologist
	Osteoporosis		For suspected stress fracture the radiograph will probably be normal and a bone scan is then required to demonstrate the abnormality	
	Bone fracture			
	EPS	Major tranquillisers	Clinical examination	Stop or decrease dose For dystonia intravenous or intramuscular antihistamine or Cogentin For other EPS oral Cogentin
	Refeeding syndrome	Probably owing to movement of potassium across cell membranes	Rule out other causes	Reassurance
	Serotonergic syndrome	Serotonin reuptake inhibitors	Physical examination Medication history	Stop serotonin reuptake inhibitors Have pharmacy check for drug interactions Symptomatic and supportive

Abbreviations: AN, anorexia nervosa; EPS, extrapyramidal syndrome.

Treatment

Treat the underlying cause.

Implications for Health Care Professionals

- Ask questions to determine what the patient means by 'aches and pains'.
- If you suspect a drug side effect or interaction, inform the physician or pharmacist as soon as possible.

Weakness

Case

A 30-year-old woman who has had AN for 14 years complains of decreased exercise tolerance. She has had excellent exercise tolerance for many years, despite AN with very low weight. She complains that for the past 2 months her ability to ride her bicycle or jog long distances has decreased. She thinks her muscles must be getting weaker, and she is concerned the weakness is due to her AN. She asks whether there is anything she can do for it to strengthen her muscles.

Comment

Weakness may be due to impaired muscle strength, early muscle fatigue, neuropathy, or reduced exercise tolerance owing to anaemia, cardiac, respiratory or deconditioning (Table 14.2). In AN, the most common causes of weakness are a proximal myopathy owing to potassium, magnesium, or phosphate deficiency, and decreased cardiovascular conditioning owing to prolonged malnutrition.

A history and physical examination should be performed to determine whether there is a specific muscle group that is weak (like foot drop owing to a compression neuropathy), proximal muscle weakness (potassium, magnesium, phosphate deficiency, selenium, hyperthyroidism), distal limb numbness (neuropathy), weakness brought on by repeated contraction of certain muscle groups that recovers after rest (myasthenia gravis), increased jugular venous pressure (congestive heart failure), or shortness of breath (respiratory muscle atrophy, aspiration pneumonia, lung abscess), or anaemia (vitamin B_{12}, folate, iron, or copper deficiency). Weakness may be difficult to demonstrate in patients who are extremely active and strong. Thus, although the patient is weaker, they may still be much stronger than the examiner.

Implications for Health Care Professionals

- Prevent nerve compression of the lateral peroneal nerve where it crosses over the neck of the fibula, of the ulnar nerve where it crosses behind the elbow (the funny bone), and of the radial nerve where it crosses behind the upper arm (Saturday night palsy) by providing soft mattresses and padding if the patient has a decreased level of consciousness. It may take 6 months or longer to recover from a compression neuropathy.
- Report shortness of breath, paroxysmal nocturnal dyspnoea, and orthopnoea as soon as they occur. In AN, these can indicate acute life-threatening disease despite the patient being young.

Table 14.2 Weakness

	Syndrome	Causes	Investigations	Comments
Muscle	Proximal myopathy	Potassium, magnesium, phosphorus, or selenium deficiency	Laboratory	Common
	Muscle fatigue with exercise	Myasthenia gravis	Edrophonium test (tensilon)	Neurological consultation
Nerve	Distal symmetrical neuropathy	Vitamin B_{12} or pyridoxine deficiency, malnutrition	Nerve conduction study	Neurological consultation
	Single nerve affected	Usually compression but can be part of an MNM syndrome	Nerve conduction study to determine prognosis and time to recovery With MNM, investigation into the specific cause of the MNM is necessary	Neurological consultation
	Nonspecific pain over one or both upper outer thighs	Meralgia paraesthetica owing to compression of the lateral cutaneous nerve of the thigh	Clinical examination	Internal medicine or neurological consultation
Decreased cardiorespiratory fitness	Cardiomyopathy	Malnutrition phosphate, selenium, thiamine, or vitamin B_{12} deficiency Valvular insufficiency	Echocardiogram Exercise stress test	Cardiology consultation
	Respiratory dysfunction	Respiratory muscle fatigue Pneumonia or lung abscess Empyema	Chest radiograph Pulmonary muscle function test	In AN, a fever may not occur in infection Respiratory muscle function tests can be ordered as part of a pulmonary function test

Abbreviations: AN, anorexia nervosa; MNM, mononeuritis multiplex.

- If the temperature is elevated above its previous level, even if it is less than 37°C, may be a febrile response to infection. This may be the earliest indicator of pneumonia or other serious infection.

Confusion

Case

Two days after being hospitalised through the emergency department for an overdose, a 24-year-old woman becomes agitated and confused. You are called by nursing staff because she is agitated.

Comment

A history and physical examination must be performed. Determine what medication(s) were taken in the overdose and what medications and intravenous fluids have been administered. Is there a history of alcoholism or recreational drug use? What observations has the nurse made?

The patient is probably suffering from an acute confusional state. The differential diagnosis includes an organic brain syndrome owing to focal or systemic cause and a functional state. The neurological examination will determine whether there are focal neurological signs. If there are, a focal neurological cause must be excluded. The focal neurological cause could be central pontine myelolysis (decreasing level of consciousness, with cranial nerve abnormalities), Wernicke's encephalopathy (nystagmus or ophthalmoplegia and ataxia), subdural (evidence of head injury, the most common is a palpable lump on the scalp), and a focal seizure. Occasionally, focal signs follow a seizure from hypoglycaemia. There are usually no focal signs.

An organic brain syndrome can occur with severe malnutrition in AN. It is often seen with very low total body fat or a body mass index of less than 10. An organic brain syndrome in AN is less likely to present with agitation, so there is probably another cause of this presentation. The most important cause to investigate immediately is hypoglycaemia.

Hypoglycaemia usually occurs in AN when blood glucose is elevated by feeding. Feeding causes an increase in insulin secretion, which moves the elevated blood glucose into cells. Why does the insulin secretion not always cause hypoglycaemia? Hypoglycaemia is prevented by the release of glucose from glycogen, the carbohydrate store in the liver. The release of glucose from glycogen is caused by glucagon, which is secreted when blood glucose levels are falling. Hypoglycaemia occurs in AN because there are no liver glycogen stores left; the tank is empty because of malnutrition

An immediate measurement of blood glucose must be performed, if the glucose if less than 2.5 mmol/L, administer 50 ml of 50 per cent dextrose in water intravenous push, followed by 100 mg of thiamine intravenously, 100 mg of thiamine intramuscularly, and an intravenous drip of 10 per cent dextrose in water at 100 ml/hour. The blood glucose must then be rechecked immediately, every hour until stable, and then every few hours. Do not stop the intravenous glucose for a at least a few days, and then only if blood glucose measurements are measured four times a day.

Other causes of confusion include alcohol withdrawal, drug withdrawal, drug interactions or drug toxicity (such as malignant neuroleptic syndrome or serotonergic syndrome), hypomagnesemia, Wernicke's encephalopathy, infection, hyponatremia, and postictal state.

Implications for Health Care Professionals

- If you notice a change in agitation or confusion, it should be reported immediately.
- Use a close observation' protocol.
- Observe for new physical signs.
- Ensure the safety of the patient.

Loss of Consciousness

Case

An 18-year-old woman with a history of AN is brought to the emergency department for an episode of loss of consciousness. She is now awake. The casualty officer asks you to assess the patient.

Comment

First, try to establish whether the patient lost consciousness. A patient who loses consciousness does not remember that which they were not aware of. So, ask them to tell you what happened sequentially. If they lost consciousness, there will be periods of time for which they have no consecutive memory.

The complaint of 'loss of consciousness' may have meant that the patient fell, was 'dizzy', felt as if they were going to lose consciousness, were very weak, felt like they were paralysed, or felt they could not breathe. The differential diagnosis of each of these problems can be quite different.

Episodes of loss of consciousness may be due to metabolic abnormalities, seizures, any cause of decreased cerebral perfusion, or trauma. In AN, the most important causes to consider are hypoglycaemia, seizures, and arrhythmia. Hypoglycaemia occurs when a decrease in the blood glucose is not corrected because the liver has no glycogen left to form glucose. Seizures can occur owing to medications or medication withdrawal, metabolic causes (hypoglycaemia, hyponatremia, hypomagnesemia, decreased cerebral perfusion, or focal or diffuse brain disease). However, unless a specific cause is confirmed, an episode of loss of consciousness should be presumed to be due to hypoglycaemia or arrhythmia. The patient should have their blood sugar monitored during cardiac monitoring, and risk factors should be investigated. Physical causes of a decreased level of consciousness include head trauma and hypothermia. Head trauma can be caused by abuse, falls owing to ataxia, weakness, or sports accidents, or they can be self-inflicted. Self-phlebotomy can cause a loss of consciousness. It almost always occurs in health care professionals. Look for a decreasing haemoglobin and unexplained needle puncture marks. Head trauma may be occult or covert. Mild hypothermia or a temperature of 36°C and above is very common in AN, particularly if the patient is wet or has been in a cold environment. However, if their core temperature is less than 36°C, they should be warmed passively; if it is below 35°C consult internal medicine, emergency, or the intensive care unit. Table 14.3 lists the causes of loss of consciousness in EDs.

Table 14.3 Loss of consciousness

	Cause	Investigations	Treatment
Metabolic	Hypoglycaemia	Blood glucose	Thiamine, glucose
	Hyponatraemia	Serum sodium	Slowly correct serum sodium and treat underlying cause
	Wernicke's encephalopathy	Neurological examination	Thiamine, and correct low magnesium or phosphorus
Cerebral hypoperfusion	Arrhythmia	Cardiac monitor	Refer to cardiologist
Seizure	Medications, metabolic causes (hypoglycaemia, hyponatraemia, hypomagnesaemia, decreased cerebral perfusion, or focal or diffuse brain abnormalities)	Laboratory Holter monitor Electroencephalogram Computed tomography Medication record	Refer to cardiologist
Physical	Head trauma	Examine the head! Computed tomography scan of head and neck	Refer to neurosurgeon
	Hypothermia	Measure core temperature (measure temperature of urine)	If less than 35°C, consult internal medicine, emergency, or the intensive care unit Rule out coexistent hypoglycaemia or drug toxicity

Implications for Health Care Professionals

- Measure blood sugar immediately on arrival.
- Administer thiamine 100 mg intravenously and 100 mg orally.
- Measure core temperature.
- Manage with patient the standard seizure precautions until another cause is diagnoses.
- Attach a cardiac monitor and record all arrhythmias.
- Remember to ask about mood, suicidal thoughts, and abuse.

Shortness of Breath

Case

A 16-year-old woman with AN develops acute shortness of breath while in hospital for refeeding. A nurse phones you to tell you the patient looks very ill.

Comment

It is likely that the patient has either aspirated her stomach contents or has gone into congestive heart failure owing to hypophosphatemia. Both situations are potentially life threatening. Severely malnourished patients with AN will usually be able to maintain their physical activity for months or years. Eventually, their exercise tolerance will gradually diminish. They will often report that this change began a few months before they present to you. This usually signals an increased risk of death from malnutrition. This is not a cause of an acute onset of shortness of breath.

However, if exercise tolerance worsens rapidly, or if it is associated with shortness of breath on exertion, then this indicates a significant abnormality usually associated with mineral deficiency and occasionally with decreased cardiac contractility. Under these circumstances, congestive heart failure may be present. The jugular venous pressure will be increased; early on, however, there may be no lung crepitations, just some delayed expiration and wheeze (so-called cardiac asthma). A chest radiograph will demonstrate pulmonary vascular redistribution, but often little else. In the setting of AN, this is a life-threatening emergency and is almost always due to severe phosphate, potassium, or magnesium deficiency. In congestive heart failure, the shortness of breath should be worsened by lying down or with any activity and relieved by sitting upright, rest, and diuresis.

In aspiration pneumonia, the chest radiograph may be normal for up to 24 hours; the more severe the aspiration, the earlier changes will become apparent. If the patient has aspirated, shortness of breath and often a dry cough will be evident. Localised dullness, crepitations, and rhonchi will be present early, and before chest radiograph changes. Leucocytosis may take a day or two to develop, and there may be no fever. Table 14.4 lists the causes of shortness of breath in EDs.

Implications for Health Care Professionals

1. Report shortness of breath, because it is potentially life-threatening.
2. Keep the patient on bed rest. Shortness of breath may be decreased by sitting upright.
3. Measure temperature, heart rate, blood pressure, and auscultate the lungs and heart.

Chest Pain

Case

A 30-year-old woman with a 15-year history of AN complains of 3 months of chest pain that is increasing in frequency. She is worried that she is going to die of a heart attack. She asks your opinion.

Table 14.4 Shortness of breath

Problem	Syndrome	Causes	Investigations
Lung	Aspiration pneumonia	Aspiration of gastric contents	Clinical examination with a high index of suspicion; the chest radiograph may be normal for first 24 hours
	Pneumonia, lung abscess or empyema	Bacterial infection Poor response to bacterial infections in anorexia nervosa	Chest radiograph
Heart	Congestive heart failure	Hypophosphataemia Less likely: low magnesium, potassium, thiamine, selenium, protein–calorie malnutrition Rarely, a myocardial infection will occur; this can occur by the age of 40 years in chronic AN	Chest radiograph Laboratory tests: phosphorus, magnesium, potassium, creatine phosphokinase A high index of suspicion for hypophosphataemia
	Arrhythmia	Decreased perfusion and increased pulmonary pressure	Electrocardiogram

Comment

AN may be associated with an early onset of atherosclerosis. In AN, myocardial infarction has been reported at an early age and 20 per cent of patients have typical or atypical angina. However, atherosclerosis does not progress more rapidly in AN, except perhaps if there is prolonged continuous amenorrhea. Angina could also be due to coronary artery spasm, severe anaemia, or an atypical presentation of one of the other chest pains.

First, take a history to determine whether the pain is angina pectoris. The diagnosis of angina is made by the history of a pain, felt as heaviness within the chest, felt in the general region of the mid chest (but always between the umbilicus and hard palate) brought on by exercise or stress and relieved by rest or nitro-glycerine. Angina lasts at least 1 minute (usually more than a few minutes) and never lasts more than 30 minutes (unless it has become a myocardial infarction).

The chest pain most commonly reported in AN is in the chest wall, is knifelike, lasts only a few seconds, and is worsened by touch. This is chest wall pain that comes from the wall of the chest, such as muscle spasm or tear, subperiosteal hematoma of a rib, or a hematoma.

Other causes of chest pain are heartburn, oesophageal spasm, oesophageal rupture, pericarditis, pneumothorax, pleurisy, pneumonia, pulmonary embolus, pancreatitis, hyperthyroidism, rib fracture, osteochondritis, self-injurious behaviour, or panic attacks. Oesophageal spasm is often confused with the pain of angina or myocardial infarction. It is usually reported as a severe heavy pain inside the chest that is not relieved by antacids. Like angina, it can be partially or completely relieved by nitro-glycerine or calcium channel blockers. Oesophageal spasm can be differentiated from angina because it is not brought on by or worsened by exercise, and it usually lasts many hours or days.

Finally, panic attacks may cause chest pain. Table 14.5 lists the causes of chest pain in EDs.

Table 14.5 Chest pain

Organ	Syndrome	Causes	Investigations
Heart	Angina or atypical angina	Atherosclerosis or coronary artery spasm	Electrocardiogram during the pain Cardiological consultation
	Pericarditis	Inflammation of the pericardium	Electrocardiogram shows generalised ST segment elevation Echocardiogram shows increased fluid in the pericardium
Chest wall	Chest wall pain related to refeeding	As for the aches and pains of the refeeding syndrome	None
	Pathologic rib fracture (a rib fracture that occurs from trauma that is insufficient normally to have caused it)	Osteomalacia Fractured ribs cause 'pleuritic' chest pain, i.e., chest pain that is severe and knifelike, and worsened by breathing	Rib fractures almost always occur owing to osteomalacia Osteomalacia is not seen in anorexia nervosa unless there is a separate cause Refer to endocrinologist
Oesophagus	Heartburn	Oesophageal reflux Vomiting	History and trial of a proton pump inhibitor, antacids, or a prokinetic agent
	Oesophagitis	Oesophageal reflux Vomiting	History and trial of a proton pump inhibitor, antacids, or a prokinetic agent
	Oesophageal spasm	Spasm of the oesophageal muscle owing to oesophageal reflux	Pain like angina, but not precipitated or changed by exertion Relieved by glyceryl trinitrate or calcium channel blockers

Implications for Health Care Professionals

- If chest pain lasts more than 1 minute, is reported to be deep in the chest, and is increased with activity, order an electrocardiogram and call the physician.
- If the patient's report of the chest pain sounds like heartburn, give 30 ml of ward stock of ward stock of an antacid. If the pain is not relieved, call the physician.

Seizures

Case

The nurse finds an 18-year-old woman with AN unconscious with tonic–clonic movements. The movements have stopped, but the patient appears to the nurse to be in a postictal state. You are called to see the patient.

Comment

If there was a loss of consciousness with movements characteristic of a seizure, then the differential diagnosis would be seizure or pseudoseizure. Pseudoseizures are associated with true seizures at least 30 per cent of the time. Be careful not to wrongly diagnose a pseudoseizure in AN. There is a tendency for physicians to favour the diagnosis of pseudoseizure in patients with a psychiatric diagnose. In AN, this mistake could threaten the life of the patient by halting the investigation of hypoglycaemia or arrhythmias.

A pseudoseizure should be suspected if there is memory of the 'seizure event' despite apparent unconsciousness during it, if the movements were atypical of seizures, if typical post-seizure confusion and tiredness are absent, if there is no change in the electroencephalogram (30 per cent of patients who have seizures have no seizure focus on the electroencephalogram, but there are nonspecific changes that last for days after any generalised seizure), and if there is absence of a normal marked postictal increase in prolactin. Table 4.1 lists the causes of seizures in EDs.

Implications for Health Care Professionals

- Check the blood sugar.
- Record observations of seizure episode in detail.
- Institute the routine seizure protocol.
- Check blood pressure, pulse rate, and rhythm.
- Check for medication errors or medications taken by the patient.
- Draw blood for serum prolactin after the seizure.

Palpitations

Case

A 17-year-old woman with AN who was admitted for refeeding complains of palpitations.

Comment

First, review the history of the 'palpitations' in detail to make sure the patient is complaining of palpitations and not chest pain, heartburn, tiredness, or muscle cramps. Then, take the history of the characteristics of an episode of the palpitations.

- Was it of sudden or slow onset?
- Was it regular or irregular?
- How long did it last?
- Did is stop suddenly or slowly?

Table 14.6 When to consult cardiology

Factors indicating need for cardiac consultation
Symptoms of faintness, loss of consciousness, chest pain, or seizure with palpitation, anginal chest pains
Resting electrocardiogram shows runs of PVB, more than 5 per minute PVB, PVB falls on downslope of T wave, abnormal site of pacemaker (not sinoatrial node), ST-T segments elevated more than 1 mm
Laboratory values: potassium less than 2.5 mmol/l, magnesium less than 0.5 mmol/l

Abbreviation: PVB, premature ventricular beats.

Determine the Pattern of the Episodes

- How many times has it happened?
- How often do they happen?
- Are they becoming more or less frequent?
- Do they seem to be related to stress, activity, purging, etc.?
- Are there any other symptoms during the palpitations, such as chest pains or faintness?
- What do you do when they occur? Do you sit down, keep on walking, hold your breath?

Palpitations are common in AN and most commonly occur after purging. The episodes usually consist of a few extra beats, the sudden onset and offset of a rapid regular heart beat (usually paroxysmal atrial tachycardia), the slow onset of a rapid heartbeat that decreases to normal slowly (sinus tachycardia after stress, exercise or purging), or the heart going fast for no reason and at other times the heart going inappropriately slowly (autonomic dysfunction). However, only an electrocardiogram can make the diagnosis of an arrhythmia, so you must record the palpitations, usually with a Holter monitor. If the palpitations cause symptoms of faintness, loss of consciousness, chest pain, or seizure, a cardiology consultation or emergency department visit must be obtained immediately, to rule out a life-threatening ventricular arrhythmia (Table 14.6).

Heart rate variability is a measure of how variable the heart rate is over periods of time. In most people, the rate does not change much, so the heart rate variability is low. If the control of heart rate is dysfunctional, which is the case when there is dysfunction of the autonomic nervous system, heart rate variability is increased. In AN, autonomic nervous system dysfunction that results in heart rate variability is often found in low weight patients before refeeding. We found evidence that ventricular arrhythmias are more likely to occur if heart rate variability is increased before refeeding in AN and then decreases over a few days to a week with refeeding. This rapid change in heart rate variability is what increases the risk of life-threatening arrhythmias in AN.

Implications for Health Care Professionals

- Monitor the patient carefully.
- Instruct the patient to lie in bed.
- Notify the physician.
- Check apical heart rate, pulse rate, rhythm, and blood pressure.
- Order an immediate electrocardiogram.

Bone Fractures

Case

A 30-year-old woman limps into the clinic. She says she cannot walk on her foot because it hurts. She wonders whether it is broken.

Comment

Osteoporosis is decreased bone mass (not decreased bone mineral density) and is common in AN. Osteoporosis, especially combined with overexercise, increases the likelihood of fractured bones. Stress fractures of the feet, legs, or pelvis; compression fractures of the spine, causing progressive and chronic pain; and fractures of the hip are most common. Weight restoration is the best way of increasing bone density in AN. The addition of graded resistance exercise, oral calcium to supplement intake of calcium to 1,500 mg of calcium a day and at least 2,000 I.U. of vitamin D_3 may help. Many patients with EDs have low total body magnesium stores. Magnesium is not only important for bone but it effects calcium homeostasis. Taking black strap molasses 15 ml one to three times a day long term is important for bone health.

Bisphosphonates can increase bone density in some patients with AN, but because taking them often decreases the motivation for weight restoration and because of their side effects, they are best reserved for patients who have worsening osteoporosis and little likelihood of ever attempting weight restoration. Oestrogen and progesterone do not increase bone density in AN.

Osteomalacia is decreased bone mineral density (not decreased bone mass). Typically, it presents with rib fractures. Osteomalacia is rare in AN because it is not caused by protein–calorie malnutrition alone. There must be another cause. It may occur to secondary hypoparathyroidism owing to chronic hypomagnesemia or hypovitaminosis D. If the patient has osteomalacia, request an endocrine consult to help identify the cause and plan treatment.

Plan of Action for the Bones in AN

In most patients with a history of AN who present with fractures and have osteopenia or osteoporosis on a dual energy x-ray absorptiometry scan – they are not weight restored. This is the problem. You must let the patient know that all of the fancy medications are going to do them no good and they are going to have lifelong pain if they do not weight restore. However, if they do weight restore, they are highly likely to gradually rebuild their bones and be free of the terrible chronic pain of the collapsing spine that one sees in older patients with AN.

Prevention of Osteoporosis

- Nourish.
- Ensure adequate calcium intake (1,500 mg/day in females).
- Ensure adequate vitamin D_3 intake (2,000 I.U. per day).

- Routine bone density scan in all patients with AN at onset of disease and at least every 2 years thereafter.
- Recommended: magnesium supplementation. Best using black strap molasses 15 ml one to three times a day.

If the Bone Density Shows Osteoporosis

- Nourish.
- Measure body fat to assess nutritional status of body.
- If you think the patient is in a healthy weight range, but they are not menstruating, then
  - Have the patient reach a total body fat of greater than 22 per cent or
  - Determine whether normal follicular development is occurring, which is evidence of normal endocrine status, on an ultrasound examination of the ovaries.
- Order serum calcium, phosphorus, magnesium, and albumen.
- Refer to an osteoporosis clinic.
- Consider use of a bisphosphonate if the osteoporosis is marked, is associated with fracture, or weight recovery is unlikely.

If the Patient Complains of Bone Pain That May Be Due to a Fracture

- Obtain an radiograph.
- If the radiograph is negative, then there may be a stress fracture. Do a nuclear medicine bone scan (not density), which will demonstrate the stress fracture.
- Consider an orthopaedic consultation.
- Measure body fat to assess nutritional status of body.

Implications for Health Care Professionals

- Instruct the patient to rest the injured part.
- Reinforce the importance of taking vitamin D and calcium.
- Explain the bone density changes that occur in AN to the patient.

Skin Rash

Case

An emaciated 23-year-old patient presents with generalised itchiness of the skin, from which she has been unable to find relief. In your examination, you note enlargement of her gums, yellowing of her palms, downy hair growth on her back, and several oddly shaped scars on her forearms and thighs. What concerns would you have regarding this patient?

Comment

Skin signs can help to make the diagnosis of AN (lanugo hair, hypercarotenaemia) and of associated behaviours such as purging (Russell's sign) or self-harm (slashing, burning,

Table 14.7 Skin rashes

Cause	Rash
Protein–calorie malnutrition	Lanugo hair Hypercarotenaemia Oedema (refeeding) Acrocyanosis Xerosis Pruritus
Nutritional deficiencies	Nail dystrophy Angular stomatitis Pellagra Acrodermatitis Scurvy Koilonychia
Behavioural	Dermatitis factitia Self-phlebotomy Self-harm
Case reports/rare associations	White dermographism Prurigo pigmentosa Pili torti Perniosis Neurofibromatosis
Purging behaviour	Russell's sign Purpura Subconjunctival haemorrhage Oedema Self-harm

and stabbing). Discussion of the skin findings in AN builds patient confidence in your expertise and helps to determine the risks of treatment (self-harm). It also helps to build rapport, because the patient will almost always accept treatment for physical complaints such as a skin rash.

Lanugo hair is diagnostic of AN. However, the reliability of the sign is not high, so that it should simply be used as a reason for a high index of suspicion of AN. Hypercarotenaemia is the yellowish skin colour (without the occurrence of yellow eyes seen in jaundice) that occurs only in AN, hypothyroidism, and in children who overeat carrots. Russell's sign is the scarring over the back of the hands that occurs if the hand is used forcefully and repeatedly in the mouth to induce vomiting. The dry and peeling skin over the palms and soles can be caused by zinc deficiency. If it is due to zinc deficiency, it will normalise in about 2 weeks with zinc treatment (50 mg of elemental zinc in zinc citrate for 3 months and then 14 mg of elemental magnesium a day if diet is inadequate). Table 14.7 describes the rashes that are associated with EDs.

Implications for Health Care Professionals

- Inspect skin the for signs of self-harm and continue to search for and document any ongoing self-harm.

- Report any new skin rash to the physician.
- Use the treatment of any skin rash to build rapport. Patients are happy to receive advice and treatment of a rash.

Amenorrhea

Case

A 17-year-old girl who is recovering from AN comes to see you in your office. She says that she is not menstruating and wonders when her menses will return.

Comment

Amenorrhea occurs at a body fat of less than 20 per cent in most females who are not taking medications that induce menstruation (oral contraceptives). With recovery of a normal total body fat, menstruation can return. Even with weight recovery, menses may not return owing to pregnancy, stress, depression, trauma, hyperprolactinemia, medications, very rare causes (like autoimmune polyglandular syndrome and hypothalamic dysfunction), or for no apparent cause. Most often, the patient has not gained sufficient weight or menses return shortly after their visit with you (tincture of time). A pelvic ultrasound examination that shows dominant (large) follicles indicates that adequate weight has been gained. It also indicates that ovulation is underway and pregnancy can occur unless contraception is used.

Important Reminders

- Pregnancy can occur without menstrual periods (as long as ovulation is occurring).
- Females are usually not aware of whether they are ovulating.
- Menstruation may not begin for 12 months after weight recovery.
- Menstruation may not return at all if severe stress or other factors that cause amenorrhea are present.

Give your patients with AN information about menstruation, ovulation, and the need for protection against pregnancy, even without menstruation, in AN.

Implications for Health Care Professionals

- Teach your patients that a healthy weight is necessary for their hormones to cycle and their bones to form.
- Ovulation and pregnancy can occur without menstruation.
- Females are usually not aware of whether they are ovulating.
- Menstruation may not start for up to 12 months after return of a healthy weight.
- Menstruation may not return if severe stress or other factors that cause amenorrhea are present.

Constipation

Case

Two weeks after being admitted for refeeding, a 27-year-old woman with AN says she has not had a bowel movement for the entire 2 weeks. She says you must do something now, because she is having severe intestinal cramps that increase each time she eats.

Comment

Common gastrointestinal abnormalities in AN include decreased food intake, decreased fluid intake, decreased or increased fibre intake, laxative abuse, vomiting, weakness of the smooth muscle of the bowel, impaired peristalsis, decreased lower oesophageal sphincter tone, impaired gastric emptying with associated early satiety, constipation, abdominal bloating, increased air swallowing, faecal impaction, and impaired recognition of need to defecate.

- Assess the causes of the obstipation.
  - Normalise the diet, including to ingest at least 2 litres of water a day (or other fluids acceptable to the dietician).
  - Check and correct dehydration, electrolytes, magnesium, and calcium.
  - A digital rectal should be performed to check for rectal prolapse and the type of stool. Usually, there is little or no rectal prolapse and there is scybalous stools (like deer stool).
  - For severe constipation involving the entire large bowel, do not use laxatives. Laxatives will cause pain and can cause perforation. Instead, use the following enemas in this order once a day: Begin with an oil retention enema having the patient hold the enema for 30 minutes, then add a saline enema with the oil retention enema, then Dulcolax microenemas, and finally soap suds enemas with 30 ml of Castile soap in 1,000–1,500 ml of water.
- Once the bowel is cleared of hard stool, use prucalopride. Prucalopride is a prokinetic agent that stimulates the parasympathetic nerves that cause the large bowel to bowel. Like domperidone and meclopromide, which affect the oesophagus, stomach, and duodenum, the mechanism of action of prucalopride strengthens the bowel, similar to the way exercise strengthens the muscles. It works the first day and the effect is usually notices over the first week or two. It should not be given before the bowel is reasonably clear of stool or the contraction will cause great pain. The dosage is 1 or 2 mg once a day. If 2 mg causes cramps, decrease the dose. Prucalopride should not be used if there is a bowel obstruction or partial obstruction.
- Bulk-forming agents bind water to give bulk and thereby help to normalise bowel function. They should be taken regularly to be effective. Dioctylsodiumsulfasuccinate, Metamucil, or similar agents are prescribed daily in conjunction with a fluid intake of at least 2 l/day.
- In addition to bulk-forming agents the following prune-based formula helps to promote normal bowel function with long-term use: Prune delight to maintain regular bowel movements:
  - Three-quarters of a cup of prunes, dates, and raisins; one-half of a cup of orange juice and one-third of a cup of water.
  - Simmer on medium low heat until consistency of jam, and mix in a food processor.
  - Dates in prune delight 20–30 Medjool dates.
- If you are concerned that you are ordering treatment that is not needed, order a plain radiograph of the bowel to assess the amount of stool, because some patients will continue to believe themselves constipated when they are not.

Implications for Health Care Professionals

- Record time and observations of bowel movements.
- Ensure adequate fluid intake.

Abuse of Laxatives, Diuretics, Diet Pills, Ipecac, and Insulin

Patients with EDs (AN and bulimia nervosa) may misuse a variety of drugs in an attempt to promote weight loss by suppressing appetite, minimising food absorption, eliminate fluid, or induce vomiting. They may abuse laxatives, enemas, suppositories, diuretics, diet pills including ephedrine, thyroid pills, herbal or other remedies with unknown constituents, or ipecac. About two-thirds of patients with bulimia nervosa use laxatives and one-third use diuretics in an attempt to augment weight loss.

Laxatives

Some patients with an ED ingest huge amounts of laxative drugs, many times in excess of the amount recommended by the manufacturer. Stimulant-type laxatives are used most frequently and are available in many over-the-counter preparations. Abuse of laxatives is not an effective method of weight loss, because weight loss occurs predominantly owing to transient loss of fluids or stool rather than prevention of calorie absorption. Furthermore, laxative use precipitates activation of the renin–angiotensin–aldosterone system and the secondary hyperaldosteronism subsequently promotes fluid retention. Chronic use of laxatives can result in serious sequelae, including loss of the normal colonic peristalsis (laxative dependency) and cathartic colon (loss of normal colon function). This results in a potentially vicious cycle of further laxative abuse. Some patients also use enemas in an attempt to lose weight. Fleet enemas or tap water enemas may be used as often as several times a week or daily. Hyponatremia can result from the frequent use of high-volume enemas because water is absorbed through the intestinal wall. Some patients spend a great deal of money on 'colonic cleansing', often citing the benefits it provides them by improving their mood. Anything that causes the bowel to dilate to cause vagal activation that may provide the improvement in mood they are referring to.

Refer to Table 13.3 for a suggested laxative withdrawal protocol.

Diuretics

Diuretics are available in a wide variety of over-the-counter formulations for treatment of premenstrual symptoms. They are used frequently in large quantities to promote weight loss. Diuretic use may begin as an attempt to control 'oedema', progressing to abuse with the ingestion of diuretics in progressively greater quantities over time. As with laxative use, the initial diuretic use may promote secondary hyperaldosteronism and reflex fluid retention when diuretics are discontinued. Instead of allowing the system to readjust and fluid balance to be restored, the patient resumes diuretic use, believing that continued diuretic use is required to control the oedema.

Patients may also abuse prescription diuretics. This is particularly common among health care workers who have access to such medications. Thiazide diuretics such as hydrochlorothiazide, loop diuretics such as furosemide, and potassium-sparing diuretics such as spironolactone and triamterene have all been used as drugs of abuse in patients with an ED. Physicians should exercise caution in prescribing these medications for at-risk individuals, especially if the reason for the drug request is vague or poorly documented.

Ipecac

Ipecac used is associated with the development of a cardiomyopathy in some patients. The cardiomyopathy seems to be reversible. It is no longer generally available.

Stimulants

Ephedrine was commonly taken to cause weight loss. Lisdexamfetamine dimesylate was initially marketed for treatment of attention deficit disorder. It is now approved for the treatment of binge eating disorder and is prescribed by some for bulimia nervosa. It is also a stimulant and being abused by patients for weight loss. If a stimulant is prescribed, it should be for short periods of time, during which weight and symptoms can be monitored. Sudden withdrawal from stimulants can cause seizures.

Insulin

Diabetic patients with EDs, particularly teenagers, may intentionally use too little insulin in an attempt to promote weight loss. This results in rapid progression of diabetic complications, including blindness and renal failure.

Superior Mesenteric Artery Syndrome

Case

You admit a 22-year-old woman to the hospital for refeeding. She has a 7-year history of AN. She recently began to lose weight quickly. When she is at the dining table with meal support she leaves the table part way through the meal and vomits as she approaches the bathroom. She says she cannot stop herself from vomiting. Some staff are concerned that she is not motivated and that she will sabotage the treatment of the other patients.

Comment

The superior mesenteric artery (SMA) syndrome is a partial bowel obstruction caused by partial obstruction of the duodenum by the SMA. The SMA and the duodenum are always side by side. Why does the SMA syndrome occur in AN? There is fatty tissue (adipose tissue) that provides padding around many of the organs in the abdomen, including between the SMA and the duodenum. With severe malnutrition, all the fat in the body decreases, including the intra-abdominal fat between the SMA and the duodenum. Once the fatty tissue that provides padding between the SMA and the duodenum is insufficient to stop the SMA from compressing the duodenum, a partial obstruction begins that limits the movement of food down the bowel.

SMA syndrome is more likely to occur when there is rapid weight loss. It can be caused by any cause of severe weight loss, like cancer. Symptoms of the SMA syndrome are early satiety, fullness, nausea, epigastric pain, and vomiting. A succussion splash, which sounds like water sloshing around in your boots, can sometimes be heard over the stomach when the patient's abdomen is moved quickly back and forth. The succession splash is caused by the excess gas, food, and fluid sloshing around in the stomach.

Voluntary emesis and decreased intestinal peristalsis are often confused with the SMA syndrome. Patients with EDs are more likely to have an unusual presentation of a common disease than a rare disease like SMA syndrome. Always consider obstruction owing to adhesions with or without torsion, pancreatitis, renal colic, biliary colic, peptic ulcer disease, and esophagitis.

The treatment for the SMA syndrome is weight gain. Providing nutrition that can pass through the narrowed section of the duodenum is the key to weight gain. This goal is best accomplished by using liquid supplements. Feeding through a nasogastric tube or a tube placed through the abdominal wall into the bowel past the narrowing by a surgeon may be necessary depending on the patient, their living circumstances, their comorbid conditions, and the cost involved. Once enough weight is gained, the tube can be removed.

The diagnosis of SMA is made by a computed tomography scan, magnetic resonance imaging, ultrasound examination, or a combination of techniques. The sensitivity and reliability of the diagnosis is highly dependent on how experienced the radiologist is making the diagnosis of SMA syndrome. Even with an experienced radiologist, there is a chance they will falsely exclude the diagnosis of SMA syndrome and a subsequent study will confirm the diagnosis.

Implications for Health Care Professionals

- The diagnosis of SMA syndrome must be considered, particularly in those patients who seem to be motivated but cannot complete their meals.
- Always exclude common causes of upper abdominal symptoms like nausea and pain before considering SMA syndrome.
- Consider SMA syndrome as a differential diagnosis of delayed gastric emptying and voluntary emesis in low weight patients.
- Use computed tomography scanning, magnetic resonance imaging, ultrasound examination, or a combination of imaging modalities to confirm.
- Weight gain will relieve the obstruction.

Rumination Disorder

Case

A 21-year-old woman with AN with bingeing and purging had a 4-year history of rumination of food. At age 17, after she began purging, she experienced worsening heartburn; later, rumination began. She said after a few bites of food, she would experience reflux, followed by an urge to burp, followed by regurgitation. She would then chew the food she had regurgitated and repeat this for hours after meals.

Comment

Rumination disorder is the regurgitation of partially digested food that is then rechewed and then swallowed or ejected by mouth. It is common in infants and persons who are mentally challenged, but is rare in healthy adults. Patients must be asked whether they have this behaviour because they will not volunteer a history of rumination. It is uncommon for rumination to be observed because patients are adept at concealing the habit.

Rumination disorder is difficult to treat successfully because the behaviour itself relieves anxiety and brings a sense of relaxation and calmness. To motivate the patient to stop rumination, discuss the marked widening of their face caused by parotid enlargement, the progressive erosion of the teeth, the diseased gums, the halitosis caused by rumination, and the fear they have of being discovered ruminating by others. Decrease stomach acid production with a proton pump inhibitor, decrease postprandial bloating with simethicone tablets, increase lower oesophageal sphincter tone with a prokinetic agent like domperidone, and correct deficiencies of zinc and iron that can cause abnormalities of eating and taste (pica and dysgeusia). Some patients will respond to chewing gum that fills the stomach with gas, or medications that decrease bingeing and purging or compulsivity.

Implications for Health Care Professionals

- You must ask each patient about ruminative behaviour because they will not volunteer the history owing to shame.
- Reduction in the severity of the ED may decrease rumination.
- Chewing gum after meals and deep breathing may help to decrease rumination.
- Rumination often begins when oesophageal reflux worsens or to relieve the discomfort of gastric fullness.

Drug Overdose

Case

An 18-year-old woman with a history of AN and major depression is brought to emergency by ambulance after her parents found her unconscious on the floor of her bedroom.

Comment

An overdose in AN should be treated like any other overdose. Certain issues, however, may require special attention.

- There are many causes of unconsciousness in AN. Therefore, rule out other causes of unconsciousness, especially hypoglycaemia, hyponatremia, seizure, and cardiac arrhythmia.
- Patients with AN often receive and stockpile numerous medications obtained from many physicians over long periods of time. It cannot be presumed that the overdose is a single drug or a recently prescribed drug.
- Coexistent vitamin and mineral deficiencies, drugs taken therapeutically, and malnutrition increase the risk of drug interactions and toxicity during treatment of the overdose.
- Calories administered intravenously, by nasogastric feeding, or orally can precipitate the refeeding syndrome.

Malnourished patients often have no liver glycogen. They are likely to develop hypoglycaemia if caloric intake (e.g., intravenous glucose) is decreased or stopped.

Respiratory support by a ventilator can rapidly decrease the serum phosphate and precipitate hypophosphatemia and death – usually beginning with heart failure. Measure the serum phosphate repeatedly and avoid hyperventilating.

- Patient with AN are likely to aspirate owing to muscle weakness, incompetent lower oesophageal sphincter, impaired intestinal peristalsis, and decreased gag reflex.

Implications for Health Care Professionals

- Obtain information from friends or relatives about drugs or medications that the patient may have kept or had access to. Patients with AN often receive, and stockpile numerous medications obtained from many physicians over long periods of time.
- Monitor the blood glucose because unconsciousness after an overdose in AN can be caused by hypoglycaemia.
- Guard against aspiration. Aspiration is likely to occur during the treatment of an overdose in patients with AN because they have incompetent lower oesophageal sphincters, impaired intestinal peristalsis and decreased gag reflex.

Compulsive Exercising

Case

A 17-year-old girl with AN has a history of extreme exercise for many hours each day. She tells you she will not be able to stop exercising in the hospital. Before she is hospitalised, she is given guidelines, among which is, 'no passes for 1 week or longer if adequate weight gain is not achieved; yoga only on the ward, once a week.'

She does not gain weight after admission. She is suspected of exercising in the shower seven times a day and running in place in her room. She is observed to be moving about on the ward constantly and she never sits still. As a result, her showers are reduced to four times a day, her door must be left open unless approved by her nurse, and her sedation will be increased until she can rest on her bed.

Comment

Her treatment is more likely to be a success if it is based on weight gain rather than on a decrease in exercise. Manualised exercise that incorporates graduated exercise that is supervised by trained staff gives the patient permission to exercise and a plan that involves gradually increasing in if there is weight gain. This increases patient satisfaction with activity and exercise without decreasing the rate of weight gain. A patient who is extremely active may need to ingest 4,500 kcal/day to gain weight. The reduction in caloric expenditure may eventually be accepted by the patient.

The patient should be encouraged to try various methods to normalise her exercise, including warming, meditation, hobbies, knitting, yoga, and reading. Explain to the patient that exercise is a good thing – but just like anything in life, too much is not good. Explain osteoporosis, muscle wasting, and chronic anorexia with a shorter life expectancy are all more likely if her exercise stops her recovery.

With successful treatment that includes weight gain and psychological therapy, exercise may decrease. It may, however, become clear that exercise is indeed an addiction. For some patients, activity to the degree that does not provide the 'rush' of aerobic exercise will be safe. In others, almost any exercise will fuel the addiction again. The treatment, like other addictions is multifaceted and involves trade-offs, monitoring, developing new powerful passions, acquiring self-esteem, and a support network.

Pregnancy

Case

A 24-year-old woman becomes pregnant while recovering from AN. Although not recovered, she is working, living with her husband, and has needed less follow-up support. She asks whether she and her baby will be healthy, whether she needs to be managed differently now that she is pregnant, and whether there are likely to be problems after delivery.

Comment

Females with AN usually experience amenorrhea unless they are on contraceptives. The amenorrhea can persist for 6 months or longer after weight recovery. Females may be ovulating even if they are not menstruating and may, therefore, be fertile without being aware of this. Most pregnancies occur before weight restoration is complete and before the patient is considered 'recovered'. Patients should be repeatedly warned to use contraception without missing pills if they do not want to become pregnant or if pregnancy is not medically advisable.

A pregnancy test should be performed as soon as pregnancy is considered possible. This should be ordered by the family physician, and consent should be obtained so that the ED clinic can be notified immediately of the results (Figure 14.1). If the patient is pregnant, the following steps are important.

- Assess the level of depression and suicidality.
- Reassess all medications, regarding their risk in pregnancy, and stop all those that should be stopped.
- Perform a thorough history, physical examination, and laboratory tests.
- The patient should be assessed and followed by an obstetrician or family doctor as a high-risk pregnancy.
- ED follow-up should be weekly for a few weeks and then reduced to monthly if the patient is stable.
- A dietician should reassess the diet and nutrient supplements.
- A psychiatric or psychological reassessment should be done, and follow-up appointments made.
- Antepartum and postpartum mothers often have great concern about the effect their ED will have on their child. Children of mothers with AN are often aware of their mother's eating habits and assume the caregiver's role to the mother within the first few years of life. Children often develop disordered eating and body image. Therefore, psychological support for the mother, and later in the context of the child or family, is imperative.

Worsening of the eating disorder in 1/3.

Chance of minimal brain damage if ongoing ketosis due to purging or starvation.

Nutrient deficiencies that impair development of the fetus.

Drug, alcohol, and medication side effects.

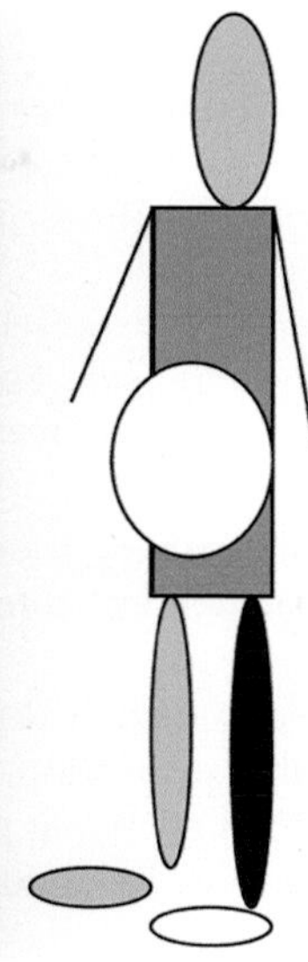

Improvement of eating disorder in 2/3.

Improvement of nutritional status of mother.

Focus less on eating disorder and more on child, life, and health.

Opportunity to re-engage in psychological therapy and family therapy.

Figure 14.1 Pregnancy

Implications for Health Care Professionals

- Most patients with AN who become pregnant do very well during pregnancy. The delivery is usually uneventful and the child is usually healthy.
- Prenatal care is usually normal with the addition of the ED care. If admission to hospital is required, it is best to admit the patient to the prenatal ward, rather than the ED ward, even if the reason for admission is difficulty eating, purging, or inadequate weight gain. The chance of success is much greater under the normalising influence of the prenatal ward. The ED team should provide specialised ED treatment on the prenatal ward.
- Mothers both antepartum and postpartum are greatly concerned about the effect their ED will have on their child. Children of mothers with AN are usually aware of their mother's eating habits and take on a caregiver's role to the mother within the first few years of life. They themselves often develop disordered eating and body image. Therefore, psychological support for the mother, and later in the context of the child or family is imperative.

Geriatrics

Case

A 72-year-old woman with a long history of AN complicated by bowel complaints and osteoporosis is sent to you for advice about her severe back pain associated with multiple compression fractures of her vertebrae.

Comment

About one-half of those suffering from AN will not recover. Of these, some will live on to old age, although rarely past their 70s. Often, such patients have adopted a very modest and rigid life style that provides them with happiness, until physical complications become incapacitating.

The most frequent long-term complication is bowel dysfunction and the most incapacitating is bone fracture and the associated pain. For specifics on the bowel and bones, see the sections on Constipation and Bone Fractures; what follows focuses on the special approach in the geriatric patient.

- Build trust and rapport in the context of clarifying what the patient's goals are. Usually, the goals are limited solely to the physical complaint at hand and do not relate to any change in eating or weight.
- Assess coexistent psychological comorbidity such as depression. The presentation of the patient is often due to the effect that depression, anxiety, or dementia has on the patient and not due to a change in the underlying physical condition.
- Perform the history, physical examination, and laboratory tests with special attention to those disorders that are more likely to occur in the older patient. Common diseases like hypothyroidism, atherosclerosis, and cancer should be considered.

Deficiencies like vitamin B_{12}, selenium, and vitamin A may take decades to occur. A prolonged increase in dietary fibre common in the elderly can cause a zinc deficiency. Stopping cow's milk ingestion, also common in the elderly, can cause vitamin D, zinc, or calcium deficiency. Decreased fresh fruit intake, because of expense, can cause a vitamin C deficiency.

- The dosage of medications must be adjusted downward in geriatric patients.
- Geriatric patients have impaired recognition of sensations like thirst and cold, and impaired physiological sensation to abnormalities like hyponatremia. Thus, dehydration, constipation, hyperthermia, hypothermia, and hyponatremia are possible.

Implications for Health Care Professionals

- The goals of treatment for geriatric patients are often focused exclusively on issues like constipation or bone pain. However, the complaint may be worse on the basis of a deficiency, psychiatric comorbidity, medication toxicity.
- Have a high index of suspicion for medication side effects.
- Geriatric patients have impaired recognition of sensations like thirst and cold. Monitor for adequate fluid intake and for hypothermia.

Males

Case

A 45-year-old male lawyer presents with incapacitating back pain. He has had AN for 20 years but continues to practice law and function well. He wants treatment for his back pain so he can continue to work.

Comment

- AN is much more common in males than admissions to an ED unit would indicate. Most males do not seek standard treatment because of the female orientation of treatment, the perception of EDs as a female illness, the concern that they will be labelled as gay, the acceptance of low body fat as normal in men, a pitifully small research information on males with EDs, and the absence of male subspecialised ED specialists.
- Tell the patient that EDs are common in men (e.g., male athletes), there are treatment facilities that have great experience will males with EDs, and EDs do not indicate sexual orientation. Having said this, there are some males, especially among teens, whose uncertainty about their sexual orientation makes it more difficult for them to access and accept therapy. Great sensitivity, acceptance, and knowledge of the issues involved are necessary to avoid irreparable damage to rapport.
- Offer the patient ED treatment in your general program. If he refuses treatment, refer him to those ED specialists who have special expertise in treating males with EDs.
- Males with AN usually want to have the shape of a weightlifter, heavily muscled, especially in the upper body. The muscles that are most important to the patient may be the 'mirror muscles'. These are the muscles that one sees in the mirror. This leads to relative underdevelopment of the antagonists of those muscles and therefore ongoing musculoskeletal pain. Determine the ideal of body image of your patient. It may require a high-protein, high-calorie diet to achieve. Accommodate, as much as possible, to the desired diet and make changes in diet only very gradually.

Implications for Health Care Professionals

- Males with AN usually idealise the body shape of a weight lifter.
- Males have the same rights to treatment as females.
- It is unethical to provide information about males that you are treating or might treat.
- The treatment team should discuss in advance the programmatic impact of a male patient. The team may unknowingly adopt a protective stance toward female patients, especially those who have been sexually abused or raped by a male. Care must be taken during these discussions to protect the confidentiality of the male patient, both within the treatment team and from other patients.

Chapter 15 Reducing Treatment Refusal and Preventing Relapse

The Patient Refuses to Be Hospitalised

Case

A 21-year-old woman with a 5-year history of anorexia nervosa (AN) continued to express her motivation for recovery. However, all ten admissions over the last 2 years had ended with early discharge from hospital. Each time, discharge followed a disagreement (such as whether she would be allowed visitors and for how long, whether she would be able to eat food from the outside, how often she could smoke cigarettes, the frequency of weighing her, and the amount of sedation she could take). Subsequently, she was only admitted electively and only after a contract was worked out and signed. The contract specified the length of admission, route of feeding, and her agreement regarding all the issues that could upset her admission.

Comment

Admissions for AN are often indelibly etched into the memory of the treating staff because of the anxiety, splitting, anger, deception, ineffectiveness, and the mental fatigue they can cause. A contract made before admission, often reached only after weeks of negotiation, is the most effective method of reducing many of these difficulties. A copy of the contract should be retained by the patient, with a copy for the team, and a copy put on the admission chart.

Implications for Health Care Professionals

- Review the contract to ensure that the treatment plan is consistent with it. Refer to the contract before you agree to a patient request to minimise the difficulties caused by ordering something that was proscribed.

Treatment Refusal

Ask your patient the following question if they cannot understand the need for compulsory treatment.

> If your best friend was depressed – and if your friend asked you to let them commit suicide – would you? I think you would try to help them!

AN decreases the patient's decision-making ability. As a consequence, physicians are ethically and legally obligated to protect patients with AN from self-harm, despite the fact that this may damage rapport in the short term. The decision of a patient with AN to commit suicide by starvation, as by other means, is caused by the disorder and will reverse with recovery. The courts require physicians to provide life-saving compulsory treatment in AN.

The regulations, laws, and methods of protection of patients with AN vary from country to country. The age of majority, the involvement of the family and the government, the role of social workers of other health care professionals, the need to report, the length of the committal, the review of committal, and even the rights and responsibilities of the treating physician vary between jurisdictions and must be ascertained locally.

Resolving Treatment Refusal

- Seek to engage in a sincere and voluntary alliance.
- Identify the reasons for refusal. The patient will often have lost hope for recovery or faith in the system of treatment. This issue should be addressed directly.
- Provide a careful explanation of treatment recommendations. This explanation may have to be given several times if the patient has impaired short-term memory.
- Be prepared for negotiation.
- Promote autonomy.
- Weigh the risks versus the benefits of treatment imposition.
- Avoid battles and scare tactics.
- Convey a balance of control versus noncontrol.
- Ensure that methods of treatment are not inherently punitive.
- Involve the family.
- Obtain ethical and legal clarification and support.
- Consider legal means of treatment imposition only when refusal is judged to constitute a serious risk to the patient.
- Consider a rehabilitation model of treatment in chronic AN.
- Conceptualise refusal/resistance as an evolutionary process.

Treatment Refusal: Decision Making

- Clinical decision analysis: Estimate the risk of the alternative decisions. The arguments for and against the need for involuntary treatment often do not take into account the likelihood of benefit accruing from instituting the treatment, perhaps the most important issue.
- Beneficence: Consider the benefits to the patient.
- Nonmaleficence: Avoid harm to the patient.
- Competence to consent to treatment: Assess the patient's mental capacity for decision making.
- The anorexic mind harbours two paradigms of existence: One that fears weight gain beyond all else, and one that wants to be healthy and happy. This situation is similar to that of a person who suffers from a phobia. Such an individual may be normal in every way – except for the phobia itself. Ask the patient whether they know someone who is phobic of something, or if they have heard of a phobia. Explain to the patient that any normal person can have a phobia, like a phobia of going outside. Tell them that the person with the fear of going outside will want to

go outside, will know that they should not be frightened of it, but will not be able to go outside anyway. Ask them whether they can see the similarity between that person and someone with AN.

The Patient Keeps Changing Their Mind: Using the Ulysses Agreement

Case

A 23-year-old woman with AN has been certified three times over the last year because of extreme weight loss causing an organic brain syndrome and hypoglycaemia. Each time, as her weight decreases, her insight diminished. After the last admission, with the patient recovered enough to have improved cognition. To avoid certification in the future, a contract was signed that set out the circumstances under which she should be readmitted to hospital. Using this contract, she receives refeeding earlier and requires only a brief admission.

Comment

The Ulysses agreement permits planning, consensus, and often improves understanding. The process of making the contract allows the patient to openly share and explain her fears.

Implications for Health Care Professionals

The Ulysses agreement is a contract that allows the patient and the treatment team to agree when treatment, usually hospitalisation, will automatically happen, without discussion at that time. It often takes a number of sessions to reach the agreement.

Section 6 Treatment

Chapter 16

Reducing the Treatment Gap by Self-Management

Many people with an eating disorder (ED) delay or fail to seek treatment. Moreover, when they overcome these obstacles evidence-based treatment might not be available. Strategies such as task sharing (involving carers or more generically trained therapists) and using technologies (books, apps, and web-based platforms) to augment/replace treatment have been developed to reduce the treatment gap. This chapter outlines the main self-management approaches for sufferers with EDs and their families. First, the rationale for using self-help approaches in EDs is addressed. Second, a description of interventions and of their clinical relevance, for both patients and their families, is provided.

The Use of Self-Help in the Treatment of EDs

Psychological interventions are the first choice in the treatment of EDs, according the National Institute for Clinical Excellence guidelines. However, they are costly, time consuming, and resource intensive. The increasing demand for psychological treatment in specialist and nonspecialist services for EDs, together with the lack of suitably trained therapists to meet this demand, lead to difficulties in providing appropriate treatment for those who seek and need help. Moreover, sufferers often have to endure lengthy waiting lists, which might decrease their already fragile motivation for treatment and discourage or delay the seeking of appropriate help. Finally, there are personal barriers, such as shame, guilt, stigma, fear of change, and failure to recognise symptoms as a problem that prevent seeking and receiving help, as well as engaging with and adhering to treatment. For example, the majority of people, particularly in late adolescence and young adulthood, are reluctant to seek help from mental health services. Particularly in EDs, those who abuse laxatives, those with current depression, and those dissatisfied with their current weight and shape tend to avoid seeking professional help.

Together, these factors contribute to the fact that many patients cannot receive an opportune treatment. This is crucial in anorexia nervosa (AN) and bulimia nervosa (BN), for which early detection and intervention are extremely important in preventing the illness from becoming chronic. There is, therefore, a pressing need to enrich and expand the types of available effective interventions, so that they meet the needs of the majority of sufferers. Self-management interventions may help to decrease the obstacles posed by limited resources and long waiting lists, and meet part of these needs by empowering patients and families in their process of recovery. They can be used, together with other treatments, for EDs, as a standalone treatment, or as a pretherapy intervention.

Self-Management Interventions, Definitions, and Modalities

Self-help interventions refers to 'the use of written materials or computer programmes, or the listening/viewing of audio/video tapes for the purpose of gaining understanding or solving problems relevant to a person's developmental or therapeutic needs'. This definition, developed by Marrs more than 10 years ago, needs to be expanded to include a range of new health technologies, such as internet-based programmes and the use of digital technology, to provide self-help programmes.

In 2003, the National Institute of Mental Health in England published an evaluation of the wide range of currently available self-help modalities, which includes the following.

- Written materials, such as books, manuals, leaflets, and workbooks: These tools are available in bookstores, libraries, internet, and health care centres. Although the offer of self-help books is vast, only cognitive–behavioural therapy (CBT)-based manuals have been evaluated. These manuals use an interactive format and include workbooks to guide the user through the material and help them to monitor their progress.
- Audio and videotapes and digital platforms: There is little evidence yet of benefit from the use of these materials. They are used as a supporting material for manual-based interventions. They may often include contributions from people who have recovered and who want to share their lived experience for the benefit of others. They might be beneficial for people who have difficulty reading and prefer using audio-visual material.
- Computer-based materials (CD-ROM, internet-based programmes), and multimedia packages (digital video devices, apps): Interest in computer administered CBT has led to the development of internet and CD-ROM packages that include video clips, self-report questionnaires, feedback, and self-monitoring of progress through different stages of the intervention. This strategy might be appropriate for those with a low level of literacy who prefer this modality to written materials and have access to a multimedia computer. There is limited evidence supporting their usefulness. However, it has been argued that computerised programmes are likely to be more effective than written materials because they are interactive, which increases their similarity to 'real' therapy.
- Self-help groups: Even though self-help groups are popular, there is little evidence of their effectiveness in mental health. Many of them are open groups, which provide support and a safe context for sufferers and families to share their experiences, but generally lack the structured intervention that is present in support groups. Some of them use supplementary self-help material, but more research is needed to clarify their role and effectiveness.

All these approaches have in common two crucial aspects: 1) they have a therapeutic objective, so they provide more than just support and, more important and 2) the individual who receives information learns how to help themselves, and is, therefore, the main agent of change. Therefore, self-help programmes provide education about their problem and the skills needed to overcome and manage their difficulties. They can give the individual a sense of control and responsibility in their own process of recovery.

Guided and Unguided Self-Help Interventions

The amount of individual effort and external assistance required by self-help interventions can be used to divide them arbitrarily into two types: 1) guided/assisted and 2) unguided/independent or pure self-help approaches. The amount of effort and assistance required by the individual in each type of interventions needs to be explained to the patient when a self-help program is recommended.

Guided/assisted self-help programmes involve a psychological intervention that requires minimal input from health professionals or paraprofessionals (e.g., assistant psychologist). The amount, frequency, and type of input varies according to the intervention, and includes different forms of contact with a health care practitioner or paraprofessional, for the purpose of providing support, encouragement, feedback, answers to questions, monitoring of progress, and appraisal of effectiveness. This monitoring allows the health carers to evaluate the need for an alternative intervention. The intervention can also be modified to fit the particular needs observed during the process. Contact between the guide and the patient may assume different formats, such as face-to-face sessions, telephone conversations, and email or other written support. Pure or unguided self-help interventions require, instead, only the use of the self-help materials, and are independent of health care contact, relying completely on individual effort. These interventions have the advantage of being easily accessible, but they may not be the best option for patients who lack motivation or self-confidence. In those cases, guided self-help programmes are preferable.

Herein, we describe the self-help programmes that have shown evidence of effectiveness for EDs and those that show promise.

Self-Help in BN and Binge EDs

The National Institute for Clinical Excellence guidelines recommend evidence-based self-help programs as the first choice for the treatment of BN and binge EDs (BEDs), which can be augmented by the use of antidepressants. This recommendation also applies to those with ED not otherwise specified, of the bulimic spectrum. Most of the manual based studies utilised were 'Overcoming binge eating' and 'Getting Better Bit(e) by Bit (e)'. However there several different forms of computerised interventions. For some cases, a combination of support by the health care provider and self-help (guided self-help) may be sufficient treatment, for most, such programmes will constitute a first step in treatment.

The interventions offer information about EDs, symptoms and consequences; CBT models to understand the relationship between diet and bingeing; training in problem solving, preventing relapses, and cognitive exercises; and behavioural experiments to manage bingeing and purging behaviour.

A specific note for BED: CBT is the most effective approach for BED, and it has been modified for self-help manual-based approaches. A number of studies have shown that CBT self-help, and particularly guided self-help programmes, are effective treatment of BED in reducing the frequency of binge eating and ED psychopathology, in specialty, but also in nonspeciality settings.

Self-Help for AN

In AN, there is less of an evidence base for self-help for the individual, although there are now several books and computerised treatments that provide information and skills to help support recovery for carers. The clinical course of AN can be protracted (over 20 years in some cases) and self-management materials could allow the patient to reinforce their learning when needed, and may be useful as a supplementary intervention in AN, providing a means of delivering psychoeducation, motivation, and self-monitoring (e.g., use of workbooks).

Self-Help for Carers

Families and other relatives are the main carers for the sufferers, even beyond adolescence. In Chapter 2 we discussed how the interpersonal dimension is one of the four core maintenance factors of EDs. This implies that an effective intervention for EDs, in most of cases, must include the family (parents, siblings, and partners). For younger adolescents, the family-based approach in which parents control eating is appropriate; however, this approach is less suitable for adults. Sharing information and advising on optimising communication and behavioural management of many of the comorbidities that accrue over course of an EDs have been found to reduce carer burden and show some benefits for people at all stages of AN.

Conclusions

Self-help interventions are very popular for treatment of EDs. They can help to address some of the unmet needs of sufferers and their families, especially those related to difficulty in accessing psychological treatments, either because services are insufficient to meet the demand or because of geographical or personal barriers to service delivery.

There is evidence for the use of self-help intervention in the treatment if EDs, especially for BN, BED, and ED not otherwise specified of the bulimic spectrum. These interventions can be used either as a standalone treatment or as a first step in the treatment of EDs. The use and delivery of self-help programmes are changing. Introducing new technologies to the development and delivery of self-help modalities (such as computer and internet-based programs, telephone, and email) may decrease the disadvantages of traditional models that require the presence of and direct contact with the heath care provider.

Implications for Health Care Professionals

- There is evidence for the use of self-help intervention in the treatment of BN, BED, and ED not otherwise specified of the bulimic spectrum.
- Self-help can also be used for carers.
- Self-help programmes require motivation and self-efficacy, as well as a certain level of literacy are necessary.
- Some self-help might be contraindicated, like weight loss self-help for those with AN.
- Self-help may be counterproductive if it extends the time before professional help is sought, if they become too reliant on it, are in denial of the illness, believe they can overcome their ED without professional help.
- Drop-outs can remain hidden if the use of self-help is not monitored by a health care practitioner.

Patient Information

- Self-help interventions are widely used and easily available in different formats, modalities, level of independency of professional care, and costs.
- People who care for you are usually desperate for accurate information about how to help. Self-help resources for them are available. (They can also indirectly help you!)
- The use of self-help interventions, including their limitations and benefits, should be discussed with your health provider. Discuss your expectations, fears, and assumptions regarding this intervention with your health care provider, before starting.

Appendix: Protocols and Algorithms

Abdominal Fullness Protocol

- Ensure the patient does not drink excess fluid before or after the meal (water load) to make themselves full or promote vomiting).
- Use warming at meal time (see Warming Protocols) to increase bowel peristalsis and relaxation.
- Prescribe domperidone or metoclopramide to help decrease early satiety, abdominal discomfort, and oesophageal reflux. Domperidone and metoclopramide 5 mg and gradually increase to 10 mg, 15–30 minutes before meals
- If early satiety is preventing intake of food and the patient cannot or will not take domperidone or metoclopramide – erythromycin can be taken twice a day in a small dose. Erythromycin can increase the QT interval so the electrocardiogram must be checked to make certain the QTc has not increased by more than 50 msec.

Important Considerations

- Rarely, domperidone or metoclopramide is used in dosages up to 20 mg, but dosages greater than 10 mg are not recommended because they are more likely to increase the QT interval on the electrocardiogram and predispose to arrhythmia. Both drugs can cause the extra pyramidal side effects of the other major tranquilisers. However, only a small amount of domperidone crosses the blood–brain barrier, so it is much less likely to cause side effects. Both drugs can cause galactorrhoea (breast milk) by increasing prolactin.

Admission Orders for Inpatient Eating Disorder Unit

- Activity – plan to encourage rest with groups, rest periods, and graded involvement in supervised activity groups like yoga. For patients with exercise addiction, further supervision may be required, including a room near the nurses' station and more frequent room checks. Warming will decrease activity for daily dry sauna or warming pad one hour three times a day will help.

> Specify limitations to activity: e.g., wheelchair only, no physical activity, no passes off the ward.

- Dietitian to order diet.

A dietitian should assess and begin feeding with 800–1,200 kcal/day. Gradually increase every few days until within 1–2 weeks the caloric content is 1,800–2,200 kcal/day, or more if required for weight gain of 1 kg a week.

- Admission laboratory work
  - Haemoglobin; white blood cell count; platelets; serum sodium, potassium, chloride, and bicarbonate; blood urea nitrogen, creatinine, aspartate transaminase, alkaline phosphatase, magnesium, calcium, phosphorus, ferritin, vitamin B_{12}; red blood cell folate; zinc; CPK, thyroid-stimulating hormone; urinalysis (midstream urine); electrocardiogram.
- Hypnotic:
  - As required: zoplicone 7.5–15.0 mg at bedtime or chloral hydrate 500–1,000 mg at bedtime, or trazodone 12.5, 25.0–50.0 mg at bedtime or clonazepam 0.5–2.0 mg at bedtime.

> Beware the habituating, amnestic, and disinhibiting effects of benzodiazepines.

- Anxiolytic
  - Lorazepam 0.5–2.0 mg sublingually up to every hour as required.
  - Quetiapine 25 mg one to four times a day as required.
  - Clonazepam 0.5–2.0 mg orally twice a day.
- Routine blood work
  - Potassium, phosphorus, and magnesium daily for 7 days and then every Monday, Wednesday, and Friday.

> Daily blood tests should be continued or restarted if there is a deficiency of any of these three minerals.

- Warming pad on medium heat one hour three times a day during meals.

Warming decreases anxiety, increases intestinal activity by stimulating the parasympathetic nervous system, and decreases non-exercise activity thermogenesis.

- Zinc citrate 50 mg of elemental zinc a day for 90 days and then 14 mg of elemental zinc a day.
- Standard supplements
  - Potassium chloride (pills, effervescent, or liquid) 24 mmol three times a day for 21 days.
  - Either sodium phosphate tablets (each tablet contains 500 mg of phosphorus) or solution (5 ml contains 550 mg) three times a day for 21 days. Continue once a day if there is continued weight gain of greater than 0.5 kg a week.
  - Multivitamin two tablets a day for 2 months and then one tablet a day. Thiamine 100 mg a day for 5 days.
  - Zinc gluconate 100 mg daily for 2 months.
- Intravenous rehydration
  - If required, give normal saline (0.9 per cent NaCl solution) at 100–150 ml per hour until intravascular volume is normalised based on the jugular venous pressure and postural blood pressure.
- Bowel routine
  - Dioctyl sodium sulphosuccinate (docusate sodium) 200 mg twice a day for 2 months or longer.
  - Give 15–30 ml of magnesium sulphate and 15–30 ml of cascara every 7 days if required for severe constipation. If this is required or if there is a history of bowel complaints, consult a pharmacist to order the bowel retraining protocol.
  - Domperidone or metoclopramide 5–20 mg one-half hour before meals (three times a day) and at bedtime.

Titrate dose upward in 5-mg increments. Use domperidone in preference to metoclopramide, which is more likely to cause extrapyramidal side effects.

Anorexia Nervosa Treatment Algorithm

Birmingham C L. Eating Disorders. *Therapeutic Choices.* Canadian Pharmaceutical Association, Canada 2017.

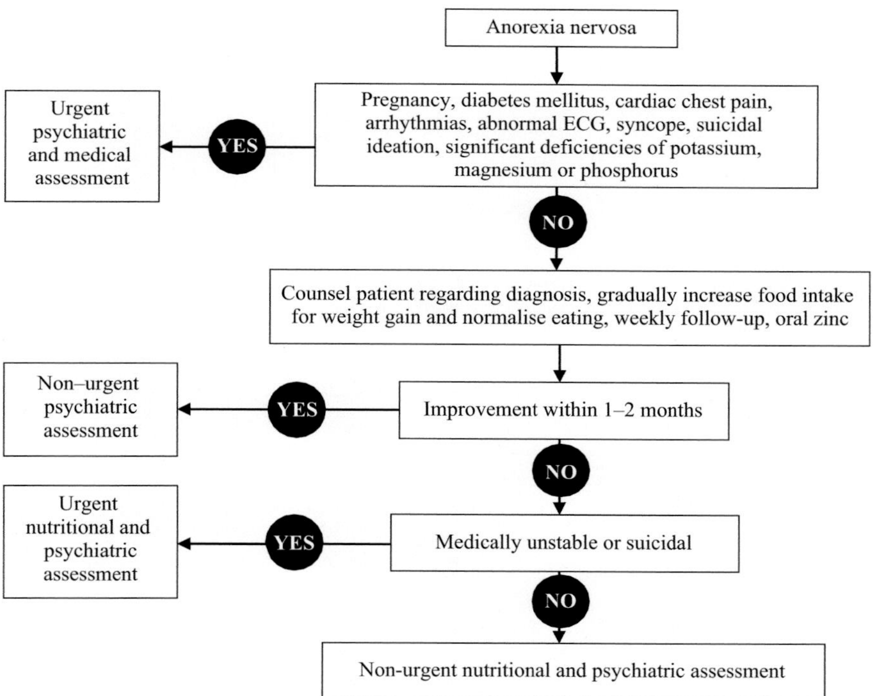

Bulimia Nervosa Treatment Algorithm

Birmingham C L. Eating Disorders. *Therapeutic Choices (5th Edition)*. Canadian Pharmaceutical Association, Canada 2017.

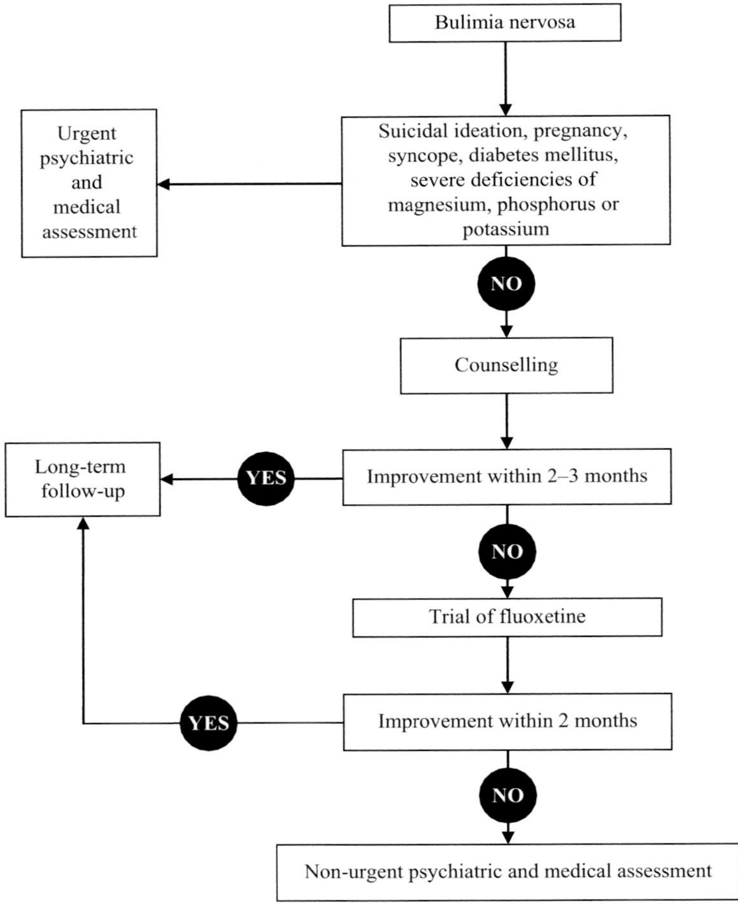

Dehydration Treatment Protocol

How to Treat

Intravenous: normal saline (0.9 per cent sodium chloride), initial bolus of 250–500 ml then 150 ml/hour until the dehydration is corrected.

Oral: if intravenous access is not available. Have the patient drink a cup of hot water with one salt cube (45 mmol of sodium per cube) three times a day. Alternatively, high-salt miso soup or oxo cubes can be used to orally replete salt and water. This is equivalent to one litre of normal saline a day.

Important

- Intravenous glucose can precipitate Wernicke's encephalopathy if there is a deficiency of thiamine, magnesium, or phosphate. Therefore, administer thiamine 100 mg intramuscularly and intravenously before giving intravenous glucose.
- Dehydrated patients have a low jugular venous pressure and/or a postural decrease in blood pressure with an increase in heart rate. Psychotropic medications may cause similar findings without volume depletion because they impair cardiovascular response due to their effect on the autonomic nervous system.

Glucagon Test Protocol

- Measure blood glucose before and 10 and 20 minutes after glucagon injection.
- Preparation: ensure intravenous access is available.
- Time: in the morning, after fasting for at least 3 or 4 hours.
- Inject glucagon 1 mg intravenously as a single push and flush through with 10 ml normal saline.
- Interpretation: a normal result is an increase in blood glucose on either subsequent reading to greater than 7 mmol/l or 2 mmol/l above the baseline to greater than 6.5 mmol/l. A lower result means there is a depletion of liver glycogen.

Important Considerations

Normal saline, not dextrose, must be used to flush the intravenous access line, the glucagon powder must be completely dissolved before administering, and the intravenous access must be completely flushed before and after the glucagon is given. Laboratory blood glucose measurement is very accurate at all levels of glucose. Needle prick measurement is not accurate when the blood glucose is less than 3 mmol/l. At a low level, needle prick glucose measurements may have an error as high as 2 mmol/l. Therefore, needle prick glucose measurement should only be used for the glucagon test.

Magnesium Intravenous Protocol and Balance Test

Magnesium Balance Test

1. Have the patient void all urine completely, then begin a 24-hour urine collection for measurement of total magnesium and creatinine content.
2. Administer 20 mmol of magnesium sulphate in 250 ml of normal saline.
3. Is the urine collection complete? Check using the total urine creatinine, which should be about 5–7 mg/day in anorexia nervosa. If it is less, the urine collection is incomplete, if it is much higher, the collection went on for too long. Either way – start again.
4. How to interpret a complete collection: if greater than 18 mmol of magnesium is in the urine, there is no deficiency (or the patient cannot absorb magnesium, which could occur with most diuretics and sometimes with protein pump inhibitor medications); if less than 16 mmol/day they are still deficient; 16–18 mmol is indeterminate.

Intravenous Magnesium to Treat Magnesium Deficiency

Administer 20 mmol of magnesium sulphate in 250 ml of normal saline over 4 hours or longer (but not faster) daily for 5–7 days. Occasionally, the infusion must be given over a longer period of time to decrease the flushing, dizziness, and diarrhoea that can occur with magnesium infusions.

Do a magnesium balance test with the last infusion to determine whether more infusions are required. If 20 mmol or more (2–4 mmol is absorbed from food every day), the patient is not deficient (unless they cannot absorb any, which is not common unless they are taking diuretics).

A low serum magnesium indicates a clinically significant total body deficiency of magnesium. Deficiency may also be present with normal serum magnesium. If there are symptoms of muscle cramps, muscle weakness, loss of visual accommodation after 15–30 minutes of reading, or impaired short-term memory, a magnesium load test should be done to test for deficiency.

Parotid Enlargement Treatment Protocol

- Warm the patient using warming jacket protocol or sauna protocol.
- Rinse their mouth with salty water several times a day.
- Rinse the mouth thoroughly after each meal. Lemon-flavoured liquid helps by increasing salivary flow. If lemon-flavoured liquid causes tooth pain owing to thinning of the enamel, do not use it.

Potassium Treatment Protocol

Normal: 3.6–4.7 mmol/l. During the weight gain phase of refeeding 20–40 mmol/day except with renal failure (increased creatinine) or increasing serum potassium.

Low: 2.5–3.6 mmol/l. Supplement with 20–60 mmol/day. Decrease the amount in renal failure.

If the serum potassium does not increase, measure the potassium concentration in a sample of urine. There should be very little potassium in the urine (a few millimoles per litre at most) when the serum potassium is low. If it is higher, the kidney is losing too much, most likely because of low magnesium or volume depletion (dehydration). Increasing the volume with normal saline or the magnesium with intravenous magnesium will correct this.

Low: 2.0–3.6 mmol/l. This requires urgent assessment and treatment. Check renal function, treat with oral potassium if the patient is able, correct dehydration (volume), do ECG and check QTc interval (should be less than 440 ms).

Very low: Less than 2.0 mmol/l. This requires emergency assessment and treatment. Check renal function, treat with intravenous potassium, correct dehydration (volume), do an electrocardiogram and check the QTc interval (should be less than 440 ms).

Elevated: greater than 5.5 mmol/l. Discontinue potassium supplementation, potassium-sparing diuretics (spironolactone, triamterene, amiloride) and potassium-containing medications (e.g., penicillin can be a potassium salt), and check renal function. Spironolactone, which may be used to treat refeeding oedema, can cause dangerous elevation of potassium if it is used in addition to potassium supplementation or in renal failure. However, elevated potassium is usually due to renal failure.

Warming Protocols

Warming Jacket Protocol

- Temperature: Warming jacket setting: medium.
- When: Preferably during meals (can be used at other times in addition, but not during sleep).
- Duration: 1 hour three times a day.

Sauna Protocol

- Measure the blood pressure (patients with a blood pressure of less than 85 mm Hg systolic should not enter the sauna because it may lower the blood pressure and cause loss of consciousness).
- Have the patient change into a hospital gown. Set the temperature in the sauna to start at 30°C (86°F) and to stop at 45°C (113°F).
- Make sure the patient consumes at least one glass of water before entering the sauna.
- Allow the patient to stay in the sauna for a maximum of 10 minutes. They may leave the door open a crack to allow for air circulation.
- When the patient exits the sauna, measure their blood pressure again.
- Instruct the individual to take a shower, during which they should gradually decrease the temperature so that it becomes room temperature. They should not to take a cold shower because this could undo the benefit of the sauna.

Index

Printed in the United States
by Baker & Taylor Publisher Services